FATHER'S HEART

LOGAN DUVALL

Published by:
Barefoot Publishing

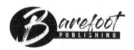

www.publishbarefoot.com

Library of Congress Cataloging-in-Publication Data:
ISBN: Perfect Bound 978-10879-766-5

Printed in the United States

Every adversity, every failure, every heartache carries with it the seed of an equal or greater benefit.

Napoleon Hill

CONTENTS

FOREWORD

From the moment I dove into Logan's manuscript for this book. I knew he had been tagged by God to be a messenger with a divine purpose. *Father's Heart* reveals exactly what the title says. In 2019, Logan Duvall got dealt a crushing blow with the cancer diagnosis of his then five-year-old boy, Lander, and his father's heart kicked in high gear to search for the optimum pathway for a cure. The reader will instantly recognizes the extent to which he has gone in devouring the research, and imparting the depth of knowledge he has gained. Adverse situations happen to us all, and with that in mind, I wholeheartedly endorse *Father's Heart* by Logan Duvall as a must-read for those searching for guidance, encouragement, and leadership in the quest for a healthier, happier, and more prosperous global community.

Martha Jordan,
Award winning author of *Let the Rivers Clap Their Hands*

PROLOGUE

One of my favorite Bible verses:

A man's heart deviseth his way: but the LORD directeth his steps.
Proverbs 16:9

It's perfect for the title of this book. God has directed the steps of my life in the most incredible ways along a path of growth through adversity.

Days come and go, weeks come and go, and months and years come and go, but it takes a concourse effort (or crossroads) to change the status quo of our lives.

We struggle through the hard times, constantly making life choices with inevitable consequences.

To see anyone suffering is difficult, but to see a loved one fighting is heart-wrenching.

As I write this, I think of the myriad ways our story could have played out up until this point. I reflect upon my walk of faith. I recall, in my darkest moment of despair, the decision I made to either turn toward or run away from God, and gratefully, I chose the former. Yet, I readily admit I am far from being a perfect Christian, much less an example of what Jesus teaches.

I continue to look to God to find strength, vowing to do my part in taking care of my son, and by using the hand we've been dealt for the highest calling. I have an unwavering appreciation for the love that God must have for all of us as our Heavenly Father. I continue to be humbled knowing He sent His own Son to die for our sins.

For God so loved the world, that he gave his only begotten Son, that whosoever believeth in him should not perish, but have everlasting life. John 3:16

There will be no browbeating or forced preaching in this book, rather *Father's Heart* is filled with the lesson of how we can sow the seeds of prosperity, and fertilize the outcome with the wisdom gained through our trials and hardships.

SECTION ONE

LanderMan

"THUMP! Thump, thump, thump…"

I held the steering wheel tightly, steadily pressed my foot on the brake, and slowly maneuvered the vibrating car to a stop along the side of the road.

A flat tire was the last thing I needed on this hectic day. I had overloaded my schedule, and to say I had a time crunch would have been a huge understatement.

I emitted a short, spontaneous sigh as I released my hands from the steering wheel and placed them on my lap.

In the seats behind me sat two of the cutest little kids; my five-year-old son, Lander, and four-year-old blonde, curly-headed daughter, Kamry.

I jumped out of the vehicle, and as they watched me put on the spare tire from the backseat window, a tiny voice pierced through the moment.

"Daddy, this is the worst day ever." It was Lander.

I cut an upwards glance at him as I tightened the lug nuts, and with a newly found, unwavering strength, replied, "No it's not. We are all alive and together. "

There was a time my day would have been ruined. However, July 13, 2019, and the word *CANCER,* forever changed my perspective on life.

The tire got changed, we came home, cooked and played outside.

Every day is a blessing. Every single day.

My Wake-Up Call from God

You live life looking forward, you understand life looking backward.
Soren Kierkegaard

My name is Logan Duvall. As I write, I'm a thirty-two-year-old small business owner living in Arkansas. I am grateful for the triumphs in my career, however, my most cherished accomplishments are, without a doubt, my four beautiful children.

I love being a parent. I love being able to look upon the countenance of a child that I had a hand in creating. The little mannerisms and facial features where I can see glimpses of myself.

Being a parent has been one of the greatest gifts of my life. Before parenthood, I didn't know what it meant to be one or how to do it. On the day, I held my firstborn child, I had to face the stark reality that I was not going to be given a handbook to prepare myself for life with kids. Like other enlightened parents before me, I learned to rely on instinct, or common sense, and if all else failed, I would often tell myself, "just do the best you can every day."

That is, until "the best you can" is not enough.

On July 13, 2019, the love that I have for my firstborn son was magnified in the grip of one moment…with one word.

That one word sent me reeling as it encircled every person standing in that room - like a tornado. Fierce and devastating, it pierced us all to the core. I looked at my little son Lander lying in the emergency room bed as my entire being was immersed in fear.

Fear of losing my precious LanderMan to *Cancer*.

The gifts of cancer were wrapped in that package of magnified love.

In turn, in that clock-stopping moment, the vast and unconditional love that I have for all my children suddenly engulfed my entire being. When you come face-to-face with the possibility of losing them, it gets your attention in a way that grips your soul and sends you straight to your knees.

It was my wake-up call from God.

I wouldn't wish it on anybody, but most assuredly, I have found the blessings. I have found the immeasurable blessings of becoming a better person through a very, very difficult situation.

By writing this book, my hope is that in sharing our experience with others, we can bless other families whose entire world has been crushed by the cataclysmic diagnosis of a life-threatening disease.

I will pass on our discoveries of tools that we have used unknowingly and knowingly, things we wish we would've known, the things we've improved, and keys that we believe will help overcome some of the obstacles that raise their ugly heads within the battle for conquering health problems.

The Derailment of Your Normal

The inevitable reality is: life will ambush us with something. I pray it's not as drastic as your child being diagnosed with cancer, or the loss of a child, but unfortunately, life is going to ambush us with something. Something is going to come and derail your normal. Whether it's a breakup, divorce, a loss of a loved one, financial crisis, illness, or tragedy - challenges and adversities come in many different forms. I believe the way we overcome adversity is through a fundamental practice, of which I am a lifetime student.

One of the greatest gifts of our experience is giving others the strength, courage, and support to succeed in their battle.

I genuinely don't think I could have handled the myriad of life's challenges in 2019 had it occurred at any other time in life. It would have been too much. Being healthy physically and mentally allowed me to heal an extensive injury and brace for the life-altering gut punch.

Adversity manifests itself in an infinite amount of ways. Mine just happened to be a severe burn, a pregnancy, a cancer diagnosis of a child, a new baby being born, running a business, being a parent of three, and juggling regular life responsibilities, while balancing relationships, all in less than a year. Adding to the craziness was being in a relatively new relationship, and spending a lot of time with my ex-wife at the hospital, who just so happened to also be pregnant. I couldn't make this up.

I wrote this book to tell our story and how I fought vigorously to save my son. I am not a doctor or a health practitioner, therefore I can't stress enough that I am not giving medical advice. I'm merely reliving and dissecting how in the world we made it to today.

In sharing my personal experience, I hope you will take away at least one thing that makes a huge difference in your life.

Weathering the Storm

It's Thanksgiving…two days out of chemo. Lander has been throwing up and wanting me to hold him. It's heartbreaking. He feels awful, and it's a reminder that our situation will be used to help others. Life indeed can be a heck of a ride.

I've wholly engrossed myself in learning to give Lander the best chance to not only beat cancer but to thrive in life. Very early on, I promised to use our experience to help others. This book is that promise coming to fruition.

If we can make it through our storm, I pray you can make it through yours. It's my deepest desire the following information gives you what you need to weather whatever storm you're going through.

He will not be afraid of evil tidings; His heart is steadfast, trusting in the LORD. Psalms 112:7

Dad, My Pee Is Orange

Being a partner in a family business has been an incredible blessing. My son and daughter, Lander and Kamry, have been able to spend much of their childhood playing outside under huge pecan trees, interacting with customers, and most importantly, spending quality time with family. Four generations are together at those times. Looking back now warms my heart and magnifies the unique opportunity.

Me & McGee Market in North Little Rock, Arkansas, was started by my maternal grandparents, Larry and Debbie McGee, and has since grown from the initial produce stand supplied by their garden, to a destination supporting many other businesses.

Lander and Kamry have spent much of their time running around playing on the swing set and digging in the dirt. All within eyeshot of the bustling little market.

July 12, 2019, started no differently than so many other days. It was hot and humid, and the kids wanted to play in the water sprinkler. They ran, screamed, and had a blast. By the end of the day, they were worn out.

By the time we got home, it was pushing 7 pm. We ate and started our nighttime routine of taking showers and getting ready for bed.

Before he climbed into his bed, my pajama-clad Lander looked up at me and said: "Dad, my pee is orange."

I looked at Amber with a confused look and walked into the bathroom. His pee was bright pink. My heart fluttered.

I had previously spent years working in EMS and had many friends who were in the medical field, including Amber's mother. I immediately began reaching out, asking opinions while I was trying to wrap my mind around the color change. We carried pickled beets and blueberries, and I thought maybe he had eaten some, but after confirming with my mom that he hadn't, I mentally crossed that off the list. I couldn't come up with anything.

Maybe it was a urinary tract infection, or perhaps even kidney stones. Lander wasn't in pain, and I made sure he had a big drink of water before he went to sleep.

I kept telling myself that it was something minor, but for a greater peace of mind, I decided to get him into the doctor first thing the next morning.

I began calling as soon as his pediatrician's office opened. The voice on the other end of the phone informed me that it was Friday, and they were out for the weekend. A nagging sense of urgency told me not to wait until Monday, so I hung up and called Arkansas Children's Hospital to get Lander into their clinic. Another stumbling block appeared. Since he wasn't already a patient, we would have to wait until after clinic hours closed to come in that afternoon.

Were we in an emergency situation? I was overcome by an overwhelming determination to have Lander seen by a doctor immediately.

I made the call to go to Arkansas Children's Hospital ER.

In less than sixteen hours from Lander initially telling me his pee was off-color, we found ourselves sitting in an ER room at Arkansas Children's Hospital.

As ER personnel hustled and bustled around my little boy, I couldn't help but wonder if I was overreacting by bypassing the clinic. The staff was great and assured me it was fine.

The first thing they did was perform a urine analysis to see if there was an infection. A while later, the results came back with no infection showing, but blood confirmed.

While we waited for more test results, Lander told me he had to go to the bathroom. I took him and when he was finished, my heart sank to the floor. There were chunks of blood in the toilet which completely freaked me out.

I hurriedly got the kids situated in the room and went to the nurses' station to tell them what I had seen in Lander's urine. Upon them hearing about the blood, and me seeing their reaction, I was instantly unnerved as I felt for the first time that we just might be in a very serious predicament.

I rushed back to Lander's room, hastily followed by ER staff. I watched with growing trepidation as I recognized the need to get IV access and fluids.

At the moment, I couldn't help but be so impressed with how the nurses treated Lander. His nurse, Randy, asked what his favorite superhero was, to which Lander replied, "Dr. Strange!" Randy then pulled up a video on his phone for Lander to watch. They successfully got the IV started on the first try. No tears, no fighting, or screaming. He was a trooper.

With Adversity Comes Strength

Lander, Kamry, and I sat in that little room for a while until my fiancé, Amber, the kids' mom, Kaitlin, and her mom, Gina showed up. He was still peeing blood.

The bloodwork came back fine and off we went to get an ultrasound. After bonding with Randy over the comic book hero, Dr. Strange, Lander wanted Randy to carry him all the way to get an ultrasound. It was a sweet moment with Lander's trust in him.

Lander and I were ushered into the dark ultrasound room as Randy placed Lander down on the bed. My mind raced.

It seemed to take forever as the ultrasound tech methodically scanned his belly and typed on her computer.

I fought the urge to ask her what she saw, at the same time knowing the universal response would be that I had to wait for the doctor. I was becoming impatient. I needed to know now.

"They should have found out something already. What is going on?" I thought to myself. As I nervously drummed my fingers on my leg, I went into full *Dad Mode*. The one-sided conversation I was having in my head brought me to terms with the truth. The reality. I knew without a doubt that whatever happened from that point going forward, I had a job to do. "I have to be calm and strong for my family. Lander and everyone back in the room will feel my energy."

With adversity, comes strength.

The ultrasound tech completed the scan, finished typing on her computer, and looked up from her work. I tried with everything in me to get some kind of reading from her face. Due to her necessary and professional approach to her job, rightfully, I got nothing.

We were systematically led back to Landers's room in the ER. By this time, we had been in the ER most of the day, and were all getting hungry. I was on the phone ordering food when I saw a group in the hall coming toward Lander's room. I quickly got off the phone without finishing the order.

I can still see the layout of the room as it will be forever etched in my mind and in my heart. Lander was lying on the bed as Kamry sat near him, playing with a phone. Amber, Kaitlin, and Gina moved to the edge of their chairs when they saw me quickly hang up the phone.

I stood facing the somber group of doctors and nurses as they quietly filed into Lander's room. It all seemed to be happening in slow motion and my heart sank as I felt the gravity of the situation when I realized the faces of this group were pretty easy to read...

The initial silence was deafening and lasted for what seemed like an eternity. His resolute voice broke the stillness. Clad in a black polo shirt, the ER doctor spoke directly to me. His words pierced through my clouded brain as we locked eyes. I focused in as he asked me, "Have you felt your son's stomach?"

My voice sounded like it came from someone else. "No." I responded. He motioned me to step toward him as he stood beside Lander's bed. He grabbed my hands, pushing them down on my son's abdomen. From behind me I heard the doctor ask, "What do you feel?"

"Something hard," I responded. "It's a mass." It took all my strength to stand upright without crumbling to my knees. I couldn't take my eyes away from his little stomach…

"Lander has a very large tumor in his left kidney." My heart again sank and I had to sit down.

Randy Was a Godsend

It was cancer. I looked at his little body, lost in the all-encompassing fear of the unknown as a gut-wrenching pain, the likes I had never known, flooded my soul.

I couldn't breathe as this was the worst moment of my life. Everything felt like it was closing in on me, like a weighted blanket, and time crashed abruptly to a full stop. I was suffocating. Was I going to lose my son?

In the midst of the emotional upheaval, another doctor stepped forward to talk to us. She said she was very sorry and that we would be admitted to the Hematology and Oncology floor of the hospital. This is a very special section of the hospital where they treat kids with cancer.

The doctors then explained that they had to do more extensive testing to find out exactly what it was, but they mentioned the possibility that it could be a Wilms tumor. We were told that the best-case scenario would be performing a surgery to remove all the tumor and follow up with chemotherapy. However, we had to continue to wait to receive all the test results back from the pathology from the biopsy.

From there, I sat in a chair and was passed to the on-duty oncologist. The oncologist told us the tumor was large and on his kidney. He reiterated the other doctors' hunch that the specific diagnosis was highly likely to be nephroblastoma, or more commonly known as Wilms. Wilms often has the tendency to spread to lungs, lymph nodes, the other kidney and brain. That was very grim news to hear, but we knew in order to be fully equipped to do full-on battle for our son's life, we had to know everything and every possible roadblock and all available treatment protocols. Dr. Bielamowicz assured us we would get through everything. He was direct, yet optimistic. We were very grateful for that glimmer of hope.

Life had taken a dramatic shift from 24 hours earlier - from playing in a sprinkler to this gut punch.

The team left the room. Soon afterward, Randy walked in and took me into the hall. He embraced me. Tears were rolling down my face as he placed his arm around my shoulders and said, "Let's get away a minute and talk."

We walked a little bit down a hall past the same nurses' station. It was not a secret that a team of oncologists had just left my little boy's room. Upon seeing us, the nurses stopped their work and looked up with a kind and caring sadness. I was numb and continued to follow Randy down the hall and through more doors to a little room.

I sat down in a chair. He pulled one over close to me as we faced each other. He leaned toward me.

"Logan, this is the time to break down. Get it out because when we leave here, you have to be the strong one for everyone back in that room." I believe it was a God thing that a man who 8 hours earlier didn't know me from Adam yet was sitting there giving me precisely what I needed. Randy was a Godsend.

The Unknowns Are Suffocating

We were then sent to a CT machine, and Lander was being so brave. The CT is a huge and intimidating machine for adults much less a 5-year-old. A CT scans your body to look inside. This would tell the doctors more information about the tumor and if there were other masses.

After the CT, we went up to the Oncology floor to rest and wait for the results of the scan and for Lander to get fluids to be hydrated.

Being told my 5-year-old son had cancer hurt so deeply. I was scared, and my heart was completely broken for my baby. The pain he was soon going to endure wasn't fair and I didn't know how I was going to handle watching him suffer. I didn't want my LanderMan to suffer.

While knowing we had a long, difficult road ahead, I had to stop and be thankful for the support that had already started flowing in from all over. I was humbled, and blessed at the same time. Prayers and help poured forth and from our first interactions with the staff at Children's, I knew healthcare-wise, we were where we needed to be for Lander's treatment journey.

Without a shadow of a doubt, the two ER nurses, Randy and Erika, had been picked by God to be there during the first steps of the process. I will never forget the genuine compassion for Lander and the much-needed embrace as we tried to grasp the shattering news.

The doctors had been incredible and we all were being treated exceptionally well. I believe in prayer, and we needed so much of it during that time in our lives. Prayer with unwavering faith that Lander would recover fully and live a long healthy life. Amen.

We vowed to use our situation to help others and become stronger. I've garnered so much experience and understanding that I know will be used to ease the lives of others.

There were so many things we didn't know at that point, but we did know Lander had a large tumor on a kidney. A multidisciplinary team of specialists were developing a plan for surgery, chemo, and other treatments.

Lander's mother, Kaitlin and I stayed the night in the room with him, still trying to wrap our minds around what was happening. Kaitlin, pregnant at the time, was very attentive and laid in bed with him. I spent a lot of time processing what had just happened.

I knew we had to stay positive and strong for Lander. He didn't understand what was going on and was occupied with a tablet computer. I remember going into the bathroom to take a shower. I turned on the water and sat down in the tub and completely broke down.

A parent's pain at that moment can't be described in words. The unknowns are suffocating.

The next day, Dr. B and another oncology doctor came to do a consultation on the scan. Down another hallway, we went to a little room with a TV and were shown the scan.

The doctors had some encouraging news, in that the right kidney was fine, however the tumor on the left kidney was very large, therefore none of the left kidney was going to be able to be saved. Next came more bad news. A tumor was found in his lung and lymph nodes surrounding his kidney. So again, my heart sank. That was not what we wanted to hear.

Let Your Mess Be Your Message

The same suffocating feelings returned when it was confirmed that the kidney cancer was in fact, Wilms. Additionally, there was a tumor on his chest as well as scans showing an anomaly in his neck.

The scan picked up what appeared to be a mass right at the point where the CT stopped, since the initial scan was ordered just for his abdomen. That was not expected.

We had been warned prior to the diagnosis that Wilms often spreads to the other kidney, lymph nodes, lungs and brain. Not a random mass in the neck. I was terrified.

From what we had been told, Wilms has a high success rate for not only remission but being cured. However, this sign didn't look like Wilms. My mind raced.

The cancer had spread, and he was considered stage 4. That took our breath away. A term that strikes fear into anyone that hears it, much less being said about your child. We had lost my grandfather a few years back from an incredibly difficult battle with cancer and it was still fresh on our minds. He was stage 4, and he suffered immensely. His battle was the family's battle and it took a toll on everyone.

Stage 4! How could my five-year-old baby be stage 4?

I worked EMS for years and all the cancer patients I had transported to Hospice were Stage 4. Their gaunt faces began flooding back to me. The frailness of their frames, the yellowness or opaqueness of their skin haunted me. Families in grief as we hauled their loved ones away to die. So many heart-wrenching times I had dealt with cancer. Now my firstborn has it.

We began seeing members of the Surgery Team. Again, we had a best-case scenario of removing the whole tumor, but they were concerned with it being so big that it might not come out. This would mean chemo to shrink it, then another surgery to remove it. The anxiety of everything was hard on everyone, but LanderMan was so strong and brave.

They scheduled surgery for Monday morning, and the long night before began.

We had many loved ones there to support us. Amber, pregnant with my third child, stayed by my side the first few days. Food was brought and love was shown by so many. We didn't know how long we would be at the hospital but were prepared to be there at least a few weeks.

I continued to have my regular shower breakdowns or go for walks around the hospital grounds to just get away. Kaitlin stayed right there with Lander, being her typical firm but nurturing self. I tried my hardest to make sure Lander only saw me as strong and that he had confident support. I don't know how well I succeeded but I sure tried. I never wanted him to think anything was wrong, just that we were in the process of getting better. There were so many thoughts and emotions. I wish I could tell you I stayed positive the whole time but that isn't the case.

I don't believe without first-hand experience, the anxiety of surgery, recovery, chemo, radiation, can indeed be understood. The road ahead appeared to be too hard to bear and the unknown excruciating. The heavy pressure pushing in from all directions and a sense of darkness truly was suffocating.

A family friend of my step dad, Steve's, is an Arkansas native, and Grammy-winning Christian singing artist. His name is Zach Williams, and his music has helped us get through some really tough times. My favorite thing from Zach is "to let your mess be your message." LanderMan agrees.

Social Media to The Rescue

I understand all too well the lack of control and helplessness as the result of what life throws at us.

The following are Facebook posts from the first part of our journey in the hope of giving more of an insight into the rawness of our experience. The blessings from a united Facebook team of prayer warriors are most certainly immeasurable. Our family highly recommends it as an avenue for spiritual and emotional support during your most difficult times, and for a rousing cheerleading team to share in the praise reports along the way.

Facebook Post July 15, 2019:

What a couple of days...
We've gone from a healthy, wild little man to being blindsided by a severe diagnosis.
The strength of Lander is awe-inspiring. I wish I was as strong as him.

The goodness in others has touched our hearts and given us support that will never be forgotten. I never quite knew the power of even the simplistic "praying for y'all" text, call or comment until we needed it. The outpouring of love is more precious than we could have dreamed. Thank you all.

Children's Hospital is amazing. I broke down over simply typing that. We are so blessed.
As a father seeing your child's situation being used to bring forth incredible testimonies of faith and praise is special. So special.

The road ahead is long and will be hard. The continued thoughts and prayers are needed.
Thank you

Facebook Post July 15, 2019- Second Post:

Update on Lander.

The left kidney and associated tumor was successfully removed. The cancer had spread to some lymph nodes in the area but were also removed.

The surgeon said the stage 3 tumor was the size of a cantaloupe and on the verge of rupturing.

We will have to wait for the test results on the specific type and the appropriate treatment.

While there has been great news, there are other very concerning spots. We just don't have all the information.

There is a lot of pain associated with the surgery and seeing him hurt has broken me. Landers strength, given the situation, is astonishing. He is my hero #LanderMan

Please continue to pray that Lander has a full recovery.

Everything has happened so fast and we have a very long journey ahead. Thank you for the support.

After the surgery, Lander was in a lot of pain. To remove the kidney the surgeon had to cut all the way across his belly. It was a very large incision. The surgeon told us even with such a large opening the tumor had to be worked out because it was even bigger. It still blows my mind that such a large tumor was in him and we didn't know. That is another thing that was consuming. How did I miss it? Was I an awful parent? We kept being reassured that these things happen all the time and it is hard to detect.

His little body in pain was hard to watch. It hurt not being able to do anything but be beside him.

He handled it well but was very nervous about moving. He had a catheter in and epidural.

We developed a way to get him out of bed. Most of the time he wanted his momma, but when it was time for something big - he wanted dad. I would come to him and put my forehead on his with my hands on his upper back. I would lean him forward with constant pressure on our heads as we got into a seated position. All the while telling him how good he was doing and that he was so strong. He was pretty good once we got there but going from laying to sitting after such a major surgery scared him.

Facebook Post July 16, 2019:

We've been surrounded by amazing people and prayers are helping.

Lander has understandably been in pain and is scared to move. Attention and adjustments have been made by the medical staff to give him as much comfort as possible.

Surgery team says everything on their end is looking good. Oncology is waiting for a definitive diagnosis to establish a chemo plan.

Pain team has been great and attentive and will take the epidural out in a day or so.

He is about to be able to start drinking liquids.

Every small step is huge to us. Thank you for the continued prayers for #LanderMan

---

Facebook Post July 17, 2019:

Landers first steps after surgery!

Being thrust into the position of being the parent of a child with cancer has caused me to realize a few things.

As I am writing this, sitting in the family room of the hematology/oncology floor, I've seen numerous kids without hair due to chemo and radiation treatment and lost-looking parents in a fog of confusion and fear.

- You absolutely cannot prepare for hearing those words of the diagnosis.
- The situation is far from unique. Childhood cancer is far more common than I realized.
- These babies have super powers. The little ones' strength exceeds anything I could have imagined.

Where there is a need, there is an opportunity. This situation has opened my eyes to a whole new world. A world full of people we can help. Every second we are learning from these experiences and we will use it to serve.

In a way, one piece of advice I try to use in assessing life is, "it's not the elephants that will get you, it's the mosquitos." Those big things we see (Elephants) and are looking for, aren't the ones that sneak up and bite you (Mosquitos).

There are so many little things associated with severe illness. Creating awareness, support and a means to deal with those things are of the utmost importance to us.

If you feel the desire to help, please consider participating in the Larry McGee Foundation #localfarmersmarketchallange2019. I truly believe supporting our community is as necessary as breathing. Being able to lean on others, and knowing the prayers are coming in, gives a positive feeling I honestly can't describe.
We got this! #StrongerTogether #LanderMan
Isaiah 41:13 For I am the LORD your God who takes hold of your right hand and says to you, Do not fear; I will help you.

My grandfather, Larry McGee passed away from cancer after a very hard battle. We had formed a nonprofit with the intent of helping the caregivers of terminally ill loved ones with cancer. Never could I have dreamed what was in store for us.

Facebook Post July 18, 2019:

Update on #LanderMan

This morning was a dream... but we are on a rollercoaster of recovery.

Lander exceeded my expectations with physical therapy this morning. He walked, kicked and threw a ball which was almost like watching a miracle.

Another huge step today was eating for the first time after surgery. He ate some bananas, green beans and applesauce.

Later he had his epidural and catheter taken out and the inevitable hurdle of overcoming the pain began.

All in all, huge steps. But watching the pain creep in is so hard to watch. The staff is amazing and they are staying on top of it the best they can but nothing is as effective as the epidural. We knew that going into it.

Please pray he gets some rest and that pathology comes back in the best, as far as cancer goes, outcome.

I genuinely cannot thank you all for the support. I don't believe I would have the strength to get through this without the prayers and positive words.

We will use our situation as a testimony and to help others. We got this!

Facebook Post July 19, 2019:

Friday Update.

I'm a little hesitant to make this post because yesterday morning was so good and the afternoon was very hard.
His strength is remarkable and it gives us strength. From a huge surgery Monday to riding a tricycle Friday...

Prayers and more prayers please for the test results to be what we expect or better. This waiting is rough but we will have answers soon.

Chemo will be rough but another step toward recovery. These challenges are opportunities to conquer and overcome! #LanderMan

We are blessed by you all! Thank you so much. The goodness in others has caused a lot of happy tears.

Facebook Post July 19, 2019:

My little miracle!

We are going home to rest for the fight ahead.

Praise God for the healing and thank you all for the prayers. I fully believe we were able to leave way sooner than anticipated because of them.

Tuesday will be the start of our next stage. Please keep Lander in your prayers.

Facebook Post July 23, 2019:

Post Appointment Update.

We still don't have pathology results but they feel that it's Wilms.

We are scheduled to be back Thursday for the pathology report, more scans and the first round of chemo. More scans are needed to make sure there isn't cancer anywhere else. Need special prayers for that too.

The removed tumor was stage 3 but since there is a spot in the lungs and lymph nodes he is considered stage 4. We were told that doesn't change the hopefulness for a cure. But hearing those words ripped my heart into pieces.

Chemo will be done at Children's and radiation at UAMS.

He will lose his hair and the side effects of chemo will be challenging and will be a long road.

His strength amazes me and he is my hero. He's had struggles but overall has been incredible. #LanderMan

It's been recommended that adults who come in contact with Lander have DTAP and Flu vaccines. With a compromised immune system, we are going to be extremely cautious.

The information we've had laid out to us is overwhelming but our support system is amazing.

Thank you for all the love and generosity. Please keep praying, they help but we have a fight on our hands and can use many more.

Facebook Post July 25, 2019:

Post First Chemo Update.

Pathology is back and they have confirmed Wilms with favorable histology. The oncologists are very optimistic about overcoming this but it's going to be a fight.

We have more scans tomorrow to check Lander's whole body.

There is a chemo plan and as of now will be weekly. Radiation at UAMS will begin next week but we don't know too much yet.

The first round of chemo was today. He did well but got sick when we got home but rebounded quickly and wanted to play the Wii.

The treatments destroy the immune system. We have to be so careful with him. Our Faith in God is Strong.

Romans 8:31...If God is for us, who can be against us?

With that said, we will not sit back believing there is nothing we can do. We will fight on every front and do everything we possibly can with our belief that God is for us.

The research and experience we go through will be shared with others. I believe we have been given this opportunity to overcome to help and inspire.

Spiritual Nutritional Emotional

Mental Environmental Homeopathic Support

These are areas we will focus on to work in conjunction with the amazing medical care of Children's.

Facebook Post July 29, 2019:

I don't know of a more flawed and imperfect Christian than myself.

Nothing will get your attention like being told your child has cancer. Everything is instantly put into a new perspective.

Lander's situation has given us all an opportunity to reflect. God will heal him completely. Those prayers are a huge factor.

I've wronged others and have been wronged, clung to my anger, and let it fester into hate.

One cannot serve God and have hate in one's heart. I've forgiven all perceived wrong done to me. I've let go of it all. It doesn't matter. The gifts I've been given will be used to serve and make a difference in the world.

As Lander's father, I must show him how to use his very special opportunity to help others. Therefore, it's my opportunity to do just that.

To be forgiven, one must forgive.

Matthew 6:14-15 New International Version (NIV) 14 For if you forgive other people when they sin against you, your heavenly Father will also forgive you. 15 But if you do not forgive others their sins, your Father will not forgive your sins.

Another big day tomorrow and more prayers are needed.
I love you all #LanderMan

Facebook Post July 30, 2019:

Radiation Consultation Update.

Today Lander had more CT scans at UAMS for the treatment plan.

He has done every single scan, even the nuclear scan, without any sedation. He has been so brave and still through every one of them.

Chemo Wednesday, Radiation Thursday, Friday and 4 times next week.

Next week will be 4 more radiation days and another chemo session Tuesday.

We are now in the beginning stages of hair loss and immune system suppression.

God has answered many prayers but we still need many more. #LanderMan is doing great and we will get through these challenges.

Thank you all for the strength you give us.

Facebook Post August 1, 2019:

Update.

Lander had his first round of radiation today. As of now, we will have 6 rounds of generalized abdominal treatments to the area: the kidney, tumor and 2 lymph nodes were removed. It's a good-sized area covering most of his belly.

Then we will have 8 localized treatments for the spot in the lung. All at UAMS. Chemo is still on a weekly basis at Children's.

Overall, Lander has handled the treatments well. We've been told that there is an accumulative effect with chemo and radiation treatments and expect the next few weeks to be harder.

The primary symptoms are him being nauseous and fatigued. Our main concern is keeping him healthy with a compromised immune system. Hand washing, germicide and masks are very important. In addition to staying clear of any one with cold or flu-like symptoms.

Our situation is unbelievably difficult but the good that is coming out of it is more than we could have ever imagined. People are wonderful. Our support is out of this world and together with God we will beat this cancer.

#LanderMan has strength that blows me away daily. So proud of our little man. Thank you all for the prayers and love.

Facebook Post August 8, 2019:

Lander has done phenomenally well with the treatments so far and Kamry was with him today for support.

We are still waiting for the results of a genetic test on the tumor. This will tell us if we need to be more aggressive with treatments. Prayers that this last test comes back favorable like the others.

Bloodwork today was perfect. He was a little dehydrated last week.

Radiation will be every day for the next few weeks. He has tolerated it very well so far.

The bravery he has displayed has been special. Accessing the port has been the roughest part on him emotionally out of everything up to this point.

Thank you all for everything. We've got this! #LanderMan #PrayersWork #GodisBigger

---

Facebook Post August 12, 2019:

Lander thinks drinking a little coffee with dad is the coolest thing ever. (It's a very small amount.)

Monday morning was round 2 of the localized radiation targeting the spot in his lung. That puts us at 8 of the scheduled 14 rounds of radiation. Lander hasn't had a lot of side effects and we count that as one of many blessings.

Tomorrow is radiation and an additional chemo drug with the regular weekly treatments.

It's a big day and prayers that his little body handles it well are appreciated. There is a chance we will be admitted at Children's.

All of the research and practices implemented are being compiled and reviewed by multiple professional disciplines. We will share everything we learn and experience in hopes of helping others.

There are so many differing opinions on every facet of health. The information out there is overwhelming. Our goal, our mission is to be as collaborative as possible, while focusing on things that have a huge upside and limited/ no risk. I never want to argue or tell anyone they are wrong and will do my own research as to what's best for my son. The only blind faith I have is in God.

If you have a cancer success story or simply advice from experience, I would love to hear it. (Sitting at UAMS this morning, I received a call of a 13-year-old pancreatic cancer survivor, and I love the stories.) We are going to fight on every front possible to help Lander.

Love you all. Thank you for the prayers. God is doing his part and we will use the situation to serve his will.

#LanderMan #BeatCancer #GodisBigger

I Am a Perpetual Student of Life

Life had been an extreme roller coaster ride leading up to Lander's diagnosis.

The path to self-improvement proved to be a massively positive decision for me. In late 2018, I began to eat clean and healthy. I started working out and in doing so, I lost a significant amount of weight and began to feel better.

I had made the conscious effort to become the best version of myself. I knew the better I was, the better father and business owner I could be.

The love of my life, Amber, had just moved to my area from around my hometown. Being former acquaintances, we hit it off immediately.

A few months into our relationship, Amber became pregnant with my third, and her first child. We announced our joyous news on April 16, 2019.

I never really became too stressed, just more focused on execution within my business and myself.

However, the elusive stress was soon about to show up in my life in a very big way. My family and I have an outdoor farmer's market in North Little Rock, Arkansas. In June, 2019, a powerful storm came through, knocking out the power. Unfortunately, when you have a lot of money tied up in perishable items in freezers and coolers, the loss of electricity is a huge deal.

Being in the produce, meats, and eggs business, and not being able to have electricity for refrigerators and freezers is a gigantic issue. The unexpected severity of the storm and the extensive damage across the area wasn't something we were prepared for at all.

After about eight hours without power, my step-dad, Steve, and I were topping off generators with gas and preparing for another night without power.

With the generator off, I proceeded to top off the tank. It was a "safety" nozzle in that the tip had to be pressed back to flow. I tried to push it and went to grab the tip when the nozzle snapped, and the almost full 5-gallon tank started gushing out. The heat emitting from the generator ignited the gasoline and the blaze exploded all around us. Steve and I were completely engulfed in flames.

I immediately took off running, trying to put out the burning gas running off my left hand. Steve quickly got the water hose and hurriedly extinguished the fire.

After it was all said and done, I had 3rd-degree burns on my left hand and less than a month later, we would have the news that rocked our collective worlds.

The backstory is fundamentally essential. The big takeaway is that during that time period, so much was thrown at me. Those listed were just the highlights, however, I stayed focused on what I could control.

I didn't waver from exercise, stayed on target with my nutrition, and immersed myself with learning everything I could about achieving optimum health, life-enhancing nutrition, and mental and spiritual wellness. I was determined to be the rock for the family and my son.

My mindset had to be strong around them. I was far from perfect and Amber helped me tremendously by being a shoulder when I needed one.

I am a perpetual student of life eager to share what I've learned.

The Unpredictable and Poignant Odyssey

Without a doubt, the most touching parts of this journey are the entries about memorable moments in this unpredictable and poignant odyssey I've been on with my LanderMan. My hope is that by sharing these stories, perhaps someone needing to lean on our experiences will find something that helps them in their battle. Our hearts and prayers go out to you all.

Lander's journey to health has been a tough road, and he has steadfastly and gallantly retained the title of Hero.

July 25, 2019 Post First Chemo Update:
"We Will Fight on Every Front"

Pathology is back and they have confirmed Wilms with favorable histology. The oncologists are very optimistic about overcoming this, but it's going to be a fight.

We have more scans tomorrow to check Lander's whole body. There is a chemo plan and as of now will be weekly. Radiation at UAMS will begin next week but we don't know much yet.

The first round of chemo was today. He did well but got sick when we got home but rebounded quickly and wanted to play the Wii.

The treatments destroy the immune system. We have to be so careful with him.

Our faith in God is Strong.

Romans 8:31…if God is for us, who can be against us?

With that said, we will not sit back believing there is nothing we can do. We will fight on every front and do everything we possibly can with our belief that God is for us.

The research and experience we go through will be shared with others. I believe we have been given this opportunity to overcome to help and inspire.

Spiritual, Nutritional, Emotional, Mental, Environmental, Homeopathic Support

These are areas we will focus on to work in conjunction with the amazing medical care of Children's.

August 16, 2019
"The Way He Looks at Me"

Lander has no treatments the next two days and gets to rest for the weekend. The last two scheduled radiation treatments are Monday and Tuesday with chemo following Tuesday's treatment.

His blood counts have been great thus far but it's expected to be low on a few key areas come Tuesday's bloodwork. Prayers for the best possible outcome.

It's so easy to get caught up with life and take so much for granted. To worry about the little things…

I'm beyond grateful that I get to spend time with my child and have the opportunity to evaluate my priorities. The way he looks at me means more than I can adequately express. Family, friends and community matter and make us human.

Although we are on a roller coaster of emotions, we are learning that every day is a blessing. Our challenges give us the opportunity to grow in all aspects. Think about what you're grateful for, fix your mind on those things and praise God for what's good in your life.

Thank you all for the strength you give us with the continued prayers and words of encouragement.

September 18, 2019
Neva Hart Collier (Logans's Mom/Lander's Nene)
"The Father He Has Become"

Yesterday was my first time to be a part of the chemo process with Lander at Children's. When we were settled in our room, I sat back out of the way, taking everything in and helped when needed. Right off, I was amazed with my son knowing answers to questions, asking the appropriate questions and assisting when Lander needed a little extra help. I am extremely proud of the father he has become.

Then there was the hard part…watching Lander go through what has become his new normal. The strength and courage I witnessed from that little boy has made me a better person today. Honestly.

Finally, the love his sister showed through the whole process gave me insight to show how strong their bond really is and will only grow stronger. I'm glad they have each other, and I'm blessed to have them. I love my people.

September 25, 2019
"The Amazing Strength of a Child"

When Lander's journey started, the feeling of doom and complete despair still haunts me. As a solemn-faced group of unknown doctors walked into our ER room on July 12th, I knew the information we were about to receive would not be good.

Your son has cancer. The worst moment of my life...I couldn't breathe. Everything felt like it was closing in on me.

Those feelings were experienced again when we confirmed the kidney cancer was Wilms, and were told he had a tumor in his chest, as well as scans showing an anomaly in his neck.

Cancer had spread and he was considered Stage 4. A term that strikes fear in anyone that hears it, much less being said about your child.

The anxiety of surgery, recovery, chemo, radiation, and on and on can't be fully grasped unless experienced. The road ahead appeared too hard to bear.
I understand all too well that lack of control and helplessness of what life throws at us. These have been the hardest times of my life, but I am so thankful for the lessons learned.

The strength of a child is one of the most amazing things.

The giving, caring nature of people is a blessing.

Whatever you're going through, take it a moment at a time and focus on the positive. You don't have to have everything figured out. A day, hour, or even a minute at a time...just try to do your best.

God uses these situations to get our attention and provides us with the opportunity to overcome and grow beyond anything we could dream.

It's our duty to make the best of whatever we go through in life and use it to help others.

Lander is in God's hands and we have full faith in a miraculous full recovery without the typical harsh side effects of treatments.

We will continue to do our part and use our experience for the betterment of others.

Thank you for your continued prayers.

October 1, 2019
"Close Your Eyes and Tell Yourself That You're Tough"

Another Tuesday at the clinic and thank God for the wonderful people at Arkansas Children's.

Blood counts were pretty good and his immune system is holding up better than expected. It's suppressed, but high enough for another round of chemo. He again has tolerated it well.

We got flu shots and it was really hard on little Kamry. She was worked up at the first mention of a shot. Lander told her to "close your eyes and tell yourself that you're tough."

Thinking about a 5-year-old giving genuine advice from his first-hand experience is heartbreaking yet inspirational. What that baby has gone through and already overcome is incredible. Hearing him say that to his sister was a really special moment.

Gut punches happen, hard times happen, terrible out of control experiences happen…

A positive attitude and faith in God to get you through the storm is the most critical component in overcoming.

When adversity strikes, take the advice of a 5-year-old fighting cancer, "Close your eyes and tell yourself that you're tough."

Thank you all for your support. Praise God for prayer after prayer that has been answered.

October 29, 2019
"God's Fingerprints"

Today was our first time going in for bloodwork and chemo following last week's news of scans showing a small spot on Lander's lung.

The effects of chemo are becoming more visible as his hair color has lightened considerably, and has begun noticeably falling out.

ANC blood counts weren't high enough to get chemo but other indicators look good. His little body gets another week of recovery, and chemo will be next week.

The spot on the lungs is in the area he received localized radiation for the initially found metastatic lesion. The new spot, we are praying and believing, is a lymph node cleaning up the damaged area.

Overall the oncologists aren't concerned in a way that alters treatments and we feel the outcome will be fine.

With that said, they are watching it closely, and Lander will have another scan much sooner than originally scheduled.

Overview:
- Low Immune System
- No Chemo This Week
- Watching Spot in Lung
- Positive Mindset

As hard as every day can be, the blessings keep coming. Lander's challenges have made us better and the fingerprints of God are all over.

Thank you for the prayers and keeping the faith with us.

November 26, 2019
"I'm Strong Like My Daddy"

Today's blood work checked out great! The chemo today, doxorubicin, will wipe his immune system completely out. Known as the "red devil" for its color and strength in side effects. It's a big one.

The next few weeks will be rough, but we will keep pushing through. Tough little man, but we have to be so careful with him.

I asked Lander last night, "How are you so strong?" He responded, "I'm strong like my daddy."

If he only knew the tears, the anxiety, the worry, the heartbreak...You find strength in faith.

I have complete faith this situation is happening with the outcome of tremendous good.

The hardships of cancer are awful, but the impact that little guy is making is beautiful. Having a front row seat is the hardest yet most amazing experience.

Thank you for the messages, prayers, love and compassion.

Thank you for your support in life. We have been able to take a box of toys every time we've gone to the clinic. Thank you all.

February 6, 2020
Neva Hart Collier (Logan's Mom/Lander's Nene) "Lander's Bond"

This morning I am reflecting on our day spent at Arkansas Children's Hospital with Lander.

Yesterday was full of hours spent having tests run to see if there were any signs of cancer in his little body, and the doctors declared February 25, 2020 that Lander was cancer free! And it happened to be Uncle Kaleb's birthday!

It has been a bittersweet road to travel on, and I can promise you we all have been changed, forever. I'm posting a sweet picture of Logan and Lander because the bond these two have is unbreakable and truly remarkable. This little guy loves his daddy beyond measure, and this daddy is the true hero in our eyes.

Giving praise to God, and giving many thanks to those who have prayed, given support and shown us so much love. We are blessed and love you all! Thank you from the bottom of my heart....

We'll never stop supporting or fighting for Lander.

March 16, 2020
"The Lord Is Close to The Brokenhearted"

When Lander was diagnosed with cancer, no words helped ease the all-encompassing fear of possibly losing my child. All the attempts were appreciated.

I have no words to ease the pain for others.

My hometown has lost two precious souls in the last few days. No words will ease their families' pain. A baby is gone. A wife, child, mother, friend is gone. Cancer and tragedy…

In times of chaos, there are many broken hearts and enough prayers cannot be said.

Love each other. Hold babies tight. Cherish every day.

Psalm 34:18
The LORD is close to the brokenhearted and saves those who are crushed in spirit.

May 20, 2020
"Lander Has Taught Me So Much"

We really don't know what is going on.

Lander's belly has been cramping and he has thrown up most everything he drinks.

Possibly a bowel obstruction or something else. He has not had a fever. Currently waiting on more bloodwork and urine labs.

He did get some rest last night.

I don't know why we are going through this but we are learning and our experience will be used to help others,

Lander has taught me so much.

We are going to keep doing our part. God will do His and we have complete faith in full healing.

May 21, 2020
"All Prayers Are Felt"

Lander is in pain from the surgery but we are managing it pretty well. In the surgery, they found that a band of scar tissue had caused a blockage. This was from the previous surgery removing his kidney and lymph nodes, with nothing we could have done to avoid it.

The surgeon said everything went really well and they didn't have to cut into his bowels. Thank God.

There was a lot of fluid in the cavity and the surgeon said it was odd. They are sending it off to be tested but felt it would be fine.

Lander's urine output has improved dramatically. Another answered prayer.

The strength this little guy displays is incredible and all the prayers were felt. We've so much to be grateful for.

We will be in the hospital for at least a few more days. (Been admitted since Monday night).

Thank you for everything.

May 22, 2020
"Lander Has Gotten Out of Bed and Walked!"

Lander got out of bed and walked! His bowels have started waking up and he is going to get to try drinking and eating.

Thank you, thank you for the prayers.

June 8, 2020
"Struggling in a Powerful Way"

Life is filled with struggles...

I had two unexpected conversations today with men I respect immensely. Both of them are older black men, one an African immigrant, and the other a retired pastor.

Both of them are strong mentally, and have an admirable degree of faith in God. We engaged in small talk for a few minutes, then I asked them both how they were doing. Next came the unexpected conversations...

The pastor had experienced a family tragedy a few days earlier and it shook him to the core. The story in itself was hard to hear. A man so used to being there for others was struggling in a powerful way.

The second conversation was the two of us just catching up, and with the current civil issues, I asked him how he was with everything going on.

Unexpectedly, he was open and honest about the strain it had on him and the experiences he had had in life, to which I cannot relate.

I grew up in a rural, white community, and I cannot relate to what these men have gone through by being black, nor the specific life hardships they are currently going through.

By the same token, they cannot relate to having a child go up against cancer. And that's ok.

My struggles in life are not more important than theirs. All I can do is love them, pray for them, and be there if they need to talk.

The other day Lander and I were driving home and Zach Williams' song "Everything Changed" came on the playlist. Lander grabbed my phone to change it. I said, "Hold on, I love this song.' He asked "Why?"

I said, "Because it reminds me of my life. When everything happened to you, I turned to Jesus and everything changed."

My six-year-old looked at me in the eyes and said, "I'm glad this happened because it made me stronger. If the devil did this to me, he has no idea what he has done."

To say the tears began to flow would be an understatement.

I shared this story with my friends today and told them I was praying for their peace. If we frame our struggles in ways of learning and service, they can be a blessing beyond measure. I never knew I'd learn so much from pain, and my child.

John 13:7
Jesus replied, "You do not realize now what I am doing, but later you will understand."

Jesus states this in regard to Peter's objection to washing his feet. I believe God has shown me in this verse to serve through adversity and not rely on our own understanding.

You never know what someone is going through in life. All we can do is be kind. Like the Roman Centurion in Luke 7, I am unworthy of Jesus, yet through faith God has answered many prayers.

Praying for peace and unity, even for things I don't understand.

SECTION 2

Principles and Mindset

LanderMan Plan of Action

The LanderMan Plan is the plan of action I outlined and our family. I implemented it for Lander upon his cancer diagnosis, to support his body recovering from surgery, to get him through chemo and radiation, and to help during the time he had a suppressed immune system. The LanderMan Plan and Moxie - The LanderMan Plan is the principle and Moxie is the mindset.

As I look back into our journey, a vital transition happened that I didn't put enough thought into at the time.

"LanderMan" principles were created and "Moxie" mindset emerged as a foundation to move forward on our path.

The grandson of a family friend owns a Fantasy Costume Party, with actors dressed as childhood heroes and princesses. Lander's second favorite superhero after Dr. Strange was Spiderman.

Spiderman came to the market to visit Lander!

The entire scenario was excellent! Spiderman showed Lander how strong he was by arm wrestling and beating him in arm wrestling — then following it up by beating me.

Next, he pulled out a special experimental serum, allegedly created by Tony Stark (Iron Man), and Bruce Banner (The Hulk), that gives superpowers to those who drink it.

After Lander smelled it, and drank it, he arm-wrestled Spiderman again and won!

This event happened only a month or so before his diagnosis. That moment, to me, was another one of many God moments in our journey. Lander would say daily, "can you believe a five-year-old beat Spiderman?" We would tell him he was a superhero and he would beam with pride and excitement.

Why do I believe this was such a big deal? Well, from that time going forward, I reminded Lander over and over again, *that he was so strong he beat Spiderman.* To him, it was real. He believed it with every part of his little body. His belief in himself, and our faith in him, gave him incredible strength. Undeniable proof that the mind is unbelievably powerful.

After reading *The Alter Ego Effect* by Todd Herman - it clicked. We unknowingly created an alter ego for Lander in LanderMan, which subconsciously gave him the strength to endure more than anyone should ever have to face. In the book, Herman discusses a conversation with the sports great, Bo Jackson, where the topic of Herman's focus of study and coaching came up. Jackson seemingly was taken back and said that "Bo Jackson" never played a down of football in his life. He also embraced an alter ego. The crazy thing about it was his alter ego was Jason, from *Friday the 13th* movie because of his constant calm demeanor, even in horrific moments. As Lander's family, our thoughts were "if a sports legend used the method to get through and succeed, so could LanderMan." (*The Alter Ego Effect* is a fantastic book that I highly recommend).

The key takeaway for us was how we wholeheartedly embraced this concept without fully understanding what we were doing. As Lander's support team, we wore motivational shirts and rubber wristbands. As I type this, I'm wearing a red wristband that says #beatcancer in bold blue letters. I even went so far as to create an illustrated, motivational comic book for Lander.

Shortly after the diagnosis and his surgery, "Spiderman" sent Lander an encouraging video telling him that he heard he was having a rough time, and then the superhero told him that everything was going to be okay. He even told Lander that Spiderman also gets sick at times. The video made my little boy's day, and gave him the encouragement to keep on pushing through the hard days. Especially the hardest days, which included the first few days after surgery. Lander experienced a lot of pain, and was very scared to move. Thankfully, within a few days, he was riding a tricycle in the playroom at Children's. He is my little superhero.

Embrace the Challenge

We are forged in the fires of adversity.
Jason Redman

When we view challenges as opportunities for monumental change, we recondition the mind to make the best of our adversities by focusing on making sure we are moving toward a place of *"better."*

I had, and still have, moments of despair. These moments are hard. By continually feeding our self-thinking we soon realize "the initial challenge is to achieve the most significant outcome, then we move ourselves beyond anything we could imagine."

Through much of Lander's treatments, he exceeded all expectations. On January 14th, he had a double round of chemotherapy; Vincristine and Doxorubicin, known as "The Red Devil," for its color and harshness. For many, the side effects are dreadful - and sadly, Lander was not an exception.

Before he was given "The Red Devil", we reminded ourselves that if all went perfectly, this was to be his last round. I had been dreading this treatment because a long-term side effect could be heart damage, on top of the short term of extreme nausea, vomiting and fatigue. Prior to the treatment, I sat down with our oncologist who is also the chief of the department. I wanted to be reassured that the rewards would far exceed the risks. He told us he felt confident that we were making the appropriate decision for Lander.

Admittedly, it would have been easier to have made the hard decisions about myself as it's a hard pill to swallow when your question is about the best interest of your child.

After our consultation with the oncologist, we prayed for wisdom and guidance, and gave the go ahead for Lander to receive the recommended chemotherapy.

It's very difficult to describe my emotions as I watched the oncology team prepare for the activation of the infusion into my child's body. I held my breath as the red fluid slowly trickled toward, and finally into, Lander's port. I found it hard to breathe as I held back my feelings of fear and trepidation.

The clock slowly ticked forward and drip by drip, we anxiously watched as the bag of liquid was finally emptied into Lander's body.

With the procedure completed, his port was de-accessed, and we started to load up to go back home. Kamry had gotten a stroller and asked to push her bubba to the car. I moved Lander to the stroller and fastened him in it. Unfortunately, that moment is when the first gag happened. I grabbed a "puke bag" and the dreaded episode commenced.

He grimaced from excruciating pain, and his belly cramped so badly. It was so hard to watch and the utter helplessness I felt was difficult to hide. I tried to console him by telling him how strong he was and that I was so glad Spiderman had given him the potion to make him even stronger. Sadly, nothing I could say held the after effects of the chemotherapy at bay.

The vomiting was relentless and he didn't want me to do anything but hold him tightly in my arms.

By this point, my heart had shattered into pieces, but I knew I had to keep it together for him and all three of my kiddos. They needed their daddy strong.

The onslaught was relentless. Lander would twist and squirm; crying from the stomach pain.

"My belly hurts, Daddy." He sobbed as he repeated it over and over. I held him and told him I loved him, and after what seemed like a very long time, he reached the point where he didn't have anything left to throw up, and became very lethargic.

I placed him in his bed and laid down beside him. In despair, as his pain continued for hours and notably worsened, I started to get scared and decided we would go to the hospital the next morning if the pain wasn't significantly better.

In trying to comfort him, I would tell him things were getting better. Again, I told him how strong he was, and we also continued to pray. We thanked God for all the blessings in our life; our home we had to live in, the family we had to love, and the strength He gave to Lander. We then asked God to make the pain go away. We asked God to let us have a great day tomorrow.

I believed God would answer our prayers.

Around two the next morning, he relaxed and fell deeply asleep. I then went to the adjacent living room to get a little rest on the couch.

I woke up and went into his room to check on him at six a.m. To my great surprise, he was sitting cross-legged on his bed.

"Hey, dad." He piped up in his chipper little voice. My heart nearly bursts with happiness. I hugged him and asked him how he felt. He said he was good and we got up to get a drink. It was the opposite of hours prior, and to me it was a miraculous change.

Sometimes the mindset is a whole lot of "letting go" and "having faith."

Little did I know that the next day would start a stretch of the worst time in my life. After a day of playing and acting like he felt great, he woke up the following morning complaining of pain in his belly.

Every ten to fifteen minutes he would scream with pain. He would cry and want me to hold him. I called the oncology department and they said to take him into the ER.

With cancer patients having suppressed immune systems, one has to be extremely careful of possible exposure to germs or some other unhealthy environmental issue. By sitting in the open lobby, Lander could potentially contract a life-threatening sickness, therefore the staff sent us to a side room. That was the second time we had been put in a side room and my memories from the last time we were there started a flood of emotions. Like clockwork, my bouts of fear would cycle through my mind. It was heartbreaking.

As we entered the room, I saw a familiar and very welcomed face. Randy was our favorite nurse and it was such a relief to see him.

The possibilities of what might be happening were very scary. A bowel obstruction, viral or bacterial infection, part of his intestines going inside themselves; none of these would be good.

After two doctors came in to see Lander, a third one came in and it was the same one from diagnosis day.

They took Lander to get an x-ray and ultrasound of his abdomen. The fear of the unknown is distressing, and my stomach was in knots. Reminders of the results of the first ultrasound, that dramatically changed our lives, kept swirling in my mind. We had gone from a healthy, active little boy to a cantaloupe-sized tumor engulfing his kidney. Nurse Randy had carried Lander to the room the first time, and there we were again; Randy and Lander heading to the x-ray department. It was all too eerily similar.

As we got to the area, anxiety was setting in like I've never felt before. We were in the exact same room with the same ultrasound technician as the first time. I was drowning in flashbacks, holding Lander tightly as his pain continued with never-ending waves of agony.

After the ultrasound and x-ray, we went back to the ER room to await results. At this point his pain had not let up. I was relieved when they finally were able to give him medicine which allowed him to doze off for a little bit.

The family members that were there on diagnosis day were unable to be with us for this appointment. Between COVID protocols at Children's Hospital and life and general, Lander and I were on our own. My fiancé, Amber, was at work, my mom had Rowan and Kamry at her house, Kaitlin, the kids' mom was at home with her infant, and her mom was working. I was alone reliving everything and trying to comfort my son.

Finally, we got some news that everything we feared was ruled out, but the x-ray showed he was extremely constipated; a common side effect of some of the chemo drugs and Zofran, the anti-nausea medication.

They felt he would get a lot of relief once he used the bathroom. Thank God, we had some answers and a plan. They were very much on the fence about admitting him, or sending him home with an intense Miralax regimen to get him to go to the bathroom. I was torn and couldn't help but feel we needed to stay, but ultimately everyone felt we should try the Miralax at home.

We went home and started what they said to do, but his pain kept getting worse. A few hours later found us at home as he began screaming and crying with pain and throwing up.

I decided to take him back to the hospital. He was admitted to 4K, which was the oncology floor. More tests, and finally a CT scan, led to Lander having to have an expedited surgery for an expected bowel obstruction from when the original tumor and kidney were removed.

Facebook Post from May 20, 2020

Due to COVID I'm alone with Lander at the hospital.
I laid Lander in the cot and they wheeled him away for surgery. This is the second time I've laid my baby down to be taken away to be operated on... it's an indescribable feeling.
I was then taken to the waiting room by one of the operating room staff. It's a pretty long walk and she asked if I was ok.
I broke down. She told me it would be ok and that even in the darkness do not give up on the Lord. We don't know what tomorrow brings but the Lord is always good.
She got me a coffee and we talked for a little bit. As she was walking away she said I'm going to be praying for you from now on and don't you forget that black lady named Rose then she just laughed as she walked away.
A little while later I sat down to text updates and Mrs. Rose came back and said I just got off and I found $10. Take it and put it in your car so you have one less thing to worry about. She said I love you and said you're going to be alright. I was bawling. Her kindness was an amazing gift. God sent an angel to comfort me ♥
Sometimes life is unbelievably difficult but the lessons we learn can be used in great ways.

Proverbs 3:5

Trust in the LORD with all your heart, and lean not on your own understanding;

I'll continue to thank God for the many blessings in my life and use what we go through to help others. God showed me again that he is always there and provided the exact comfort I needed.

In the surgery, they found a band of scar tissue causing a blockage. It was from the previous surgery to remove his kidney and lymph nodes. It was an unavoidable situation.

The strength this little guy displays is incredible, and all the prayers were felt. We've so much to be grateful for.

Writing this section almost a year after still brings back strong emotions. This was the most difficult thing I've ever experienced.

Remembering everything Lander has gone through is tough. The trust Lander had in me, and to have to hold him down while a tube was run up his nose, still gives me chills. He begged and begged to have it removed. It was horrible.

I hate that he experienced any of it, however, it gave us such insight, and the tribulations made us look toward God.

Hebrews 11:1 King James Version (KJV)

Now faith is the substance of things hoped for, the evidence of things not seen.

The Moxie Mindset

Merriam Webster defines Moxie as
  1: ENERGY, PEP
  2: COURAGE, DETERMINATION
  3: KNOW-HOW

Lander has definitely exemplified moxie, and it's after him that I name our lifestyle and mindset.

I do not claim to be an expert and I certainly didn't have a plan mapped out to get us through our ordeal. Honestly, I was taking it a day at a time. I relied heavily on past experiences, gut feeling, and faith. I'm able to look back and examine what worked and what didn't. I can highlight the things that benefited our cause, and try to help others going through similar challenges. My hope is that we can help equip others with the ability to handle life in ways I never could have dreamed possible.

> *Ask and it will be given to you; seek and you will*
> *find; knock and the door will be opened to you.*
> Mathew 7:7

Moxie Creed:

To live our lives to the fullest, we must control our mindsets, maximize our health, and cultivate our energy.

Living our lives to the fullest means we must navigate our way through the ups and downs. Getting through starts with self. Let's build ourselves to be difference-makers in this world.

Moxie Mindset:

Moxie is a lifestyle that sets us up to overcome and succeed in life. I break it down into three broad areas of focus, with subcategories: Mind, Body, Practice. All three are infinitely connected, but I break them down to establish actionable, defined steps.

"Here I stand on the shoulders of giants in their fields of study or areas of dedication in life. To use their lessons to relay to others a compilation of tactics for a better life."

Mindset:

With every adversity comes the seed of an
equal or greater opportunity
Napoleon Hill

Be not deceived; God is not mocked: for whatsoever
a man soweth, that shall he also reap.
Galatians 6:7

Our mindset is the foundational component of everything.

Framing our perspective is essential to our plan of attack. Looking back now, I can see that Lander's diagnosis brought me to a crossroad. I could have chosen to accept a terrible situation and remain helpless; it takes no effort to be a victim. To the contrary, it takes tremendous effort to identify the positive and focus on it, especially with all of the unknowns.

Desire is the seed that leads to following through, and to the dedication needed for high achievement. The beautiful thing about this approach is by making ourselves better; we can serve those around us and make a more significant impact. The dividends of being our best are more than most can imagine.

When you have a purpose supported by a deep burning desire, you can accomplish anything.

With that said, there are a lot of interrelated components to what I'm saying about a Moxie Mindset.

I'd like to tie all of this together from the wisdom of Bill Bartmann in the stages of misfortune.

- Distress
- Appreciation
- New Perspective

> *You have power over your mind - not outside events.*
> *Realize this, and you will find strength.*
> *Marcus Aurelius*

Moxie Mindset Resources:

- *The Bible*
- *Warriors Guide to Overcome* Jason Redman
- *Athletes Guide to Relentless* by Tim Grover
- *Still in the Game* Devon Still
- *Parents Guide to Warrior Mom* JJ Virgin
- *Embrace an Alter Ego* Todd Herman

Gratitude:

So much of the core of a Moxie Mindset is gratitude. There is a direct correlation with the degree of gratitude we have for the quality of our mindset. I've come to terms with the inevitability of how an ambush can disrupt your life. Without a doubt, I've experienced more than my fair share.

A life ambush can manifest in many ways - divorce, sickness, loss of a loved one, business failure, financial mishap, or tragedy.

For me, Lander's cancer diagnosis is the most recent. It fully embodied the definition of a life ambush; a life-altering moment or circumstance one is unable to prepare for.

By the grace of God, I had already committed to strengthening myself before my baby began his great fight. I don't believe I could have handled this situation at any other point in my life.

I began exercising, and strengthening my mind through reading and positivity. I dove back into healthy living and developed a dietary plan to follow. In every way, I was looking for knowledge and practices to better myself. My affirmation that the cycle of feeling better leads to working harder and feeling better.

Shortly before, my most significant life ambush to date was an accident that burnt me pretty severely. Looking back, the pain was awful, but the challenge prepared my mind further for what was looming on the horizon. I now attribute that accident to have been a powerful blessing that taught me strength and perseverance for what was to come.

We choose how to proceed after a life ambush. We are in complete control of our reaction.

Common reactions to a Life Ambush:
- Defeat us
- Define us
- Launch us

Admittedly, for most of my life, my child's life-altering cancer diagnosis probably would have defeated me. The suffering of a child hurts in indescribable ways, yet cancer has launched me into the service of others. I want to share the knowledge I've gained and practiced in hopes of sharing tools and encouragement. The choice going forward is ours.

Let's face it, life ambushes are going to happen to every single one of us. They are easier to handle when we are physically and mentally preparing ourselves.

If you're already in an ambush, take a deep breath. Ask yourself, "what parts of this do I have control over?"

Once identified, get to work on improving them. Let go of everything else about the ambush. We only have a certain amount of energy to expend. Choose what gets it wisely.

Find one thing positive in the ambush and focus on it. Be grateful for the good as gratitude is a seed of perseverance and prosperity.

As for me, I focus on the time I have with my son, on getting to love him in this storm of life. With a newfound appreciation for quality time with my children, I am grateful beyond measure.

If I chose to embrace negativity or sorrow, I would lose sight of the blessings. I wouldn't have the energy to strengthen myself and find answers to help him.

Every day I wake up and go to bed with gratitude. It has changed my life, helping me focus on the good. I have found that a gratitude journal is a fantastic tool to aid in keeping me focused on the positive things in life.

Gratitude is the healthiest of all human emotions. The more you express gratitude for what you have, the more likely you will have even more to express gratitude for. Zig Ziglar

---

Forgiveness:

Do you have any regrets from bad decisions you've made? Do you harbor anger, or even hatred in your heart for the wrong done by others? If you were being honest, the answer would most likely be yes. This isn't something to be ashamed of or hide. It means you've lived. You've experienced pain and disappointment.

When we let it, pain teaches us more than anything else. On the flip side, it can build and fester into an all-consuming black hole of negativity.

Forgiveness may seem out of place, but it was one of the most freeing things I've ever done. Looking at my son changed everything. I had lots of hate built up in my heart from the perceived wrong done to me. The dynamic of having an estranged father and son relationship hurt. Years of bad feelings were like little seeds of pain. Those seeds grew into weeds of negativity and hate. I always swore to make sure I approached things differently with my kids and their mother.

I can hear it now, "But that's easy for you to say. You don't know what I've been through." While I haven't been through the exact situation you've been through, I can assure you, I've been through a lot.

I've spent the vast majority of my life in an estranged relationship with my father. I essentially grew up without a father figure of note and I held onto a lot of hate. My mother had just graduated from high school and my father was two years older. They were kids and I can't imagine being a parent that young. My dad was in and out of my life early on for various reasons. There were a lot of poor decisions made on all sides and I always felt I had been put in a position where I had to choose between parents. With the choice being between a constant, my mother, or an in-and-out father, there really wasn't a choice as to whose side I was on. My mother is an amazing woman and has worked her butt off to give me everything she could.

For many years I hated that man, and the more I hated him the more it consumed me. I found myself being pissed off as I sat in a hospital room looking at my baby boy, who was facing a hell of a road with cancer. I was so mad that my father was coming to see him. Let that sink in. He was coming to see my sick son, and I'm mad because I was still holding on to disappointment and hurt from the past. After throwing a little fit, (I'm far from perfect), Lander's mom basically told me to get over myself and keep my mouth shut.

My absentee father came into Lander's hospital room. I sat across the room as he pulled up a chair to see Lander. He loved his grandson. It was evident in his eyes. My anger didn't go away, but it caused me to swallow my pride. Upon self-reflection, I couldn't help but feel extremely disappointed in myself. My little son was in a fight for his life and I'm mad about things that happened in the past. How did this serve Lander? The easy answer was that it didn't and by hurting myself with hate, I was hurting my son.

Forgiveness isn't just about forgiving others, it's about forgiving yourself. I love the irony in that "give" is in the word "forgive." It is the greatest gift I've ever received or given.

In an instant, I let it all go because at the end of the day, what did the past matter? Like anchors on the soul, hate destroys us by not allowing us to move forward.

As Lander's father, I must show him how to use his extraordinary opportunity to help others. Therefore, it's my opportunity to do just that.

To be forgiven, one must forgive.

Matthew 6:14-15 New International Version (NIV) 14 For if you forgive other people when they sin against you, your heavenly Father will also forgive you. 15 But if you do not forgive others their sins, your Father will not forgive your sins.

Another big day tomorrow and more prayers are needed.

Forgiving made a life-changing impact on me, and by sharing my story, I gave others a push to do it for themselves. It was beautiful.

I, like so many others, held onto the pain of the past. When you have something as drastic as your child being diagnosed with cancer, your perspective completely changes. I often tell people that the things I was stressed out about on "Thursday" didn't even matter on "Friday."

We all have reasons to be upset, but harboring that hate in your heart only hurts yourself. It grows and festers in ways that are damning. I quickly came to terms that if my focus was to save Lander, and give him the best quality of life, I could not have hate in my heart.

I learned that in moments of despair, a person will do anything. I prayed for God to forgive me. I prayed for God to not hold my sins against my children. I also asked Him not to hold the sins of our forefathers against Lander.

I know too many this will sound outlandish, but it was the most freeing thing I have ever done. I completely let go of every single ounce of hate I had in my heart, in an instant. For many years I had held onto an all-consuming burning hatred for a few people that had hurt or disappointed me. By praying for forgiveness (for them and for myself), I let it all go. It is the best thing I've ever done.

Let me clarify something about the prior paragraph. Forgiveness of others does not always mean that those I forgave will be back in my life, or that I have forgotten the past. Acceptance is another way to accurately describe what I embraced. I've been burnt and I know how that feels. I will not touch the fire again.

How I forgave:
1. Took ownership of the pain.
2. Let go of the anger and hatred.

Examples of Moxie:

Due to a large number of phenomenal individuals who have displayed Moxie in life, it pains me in having to leave so many out who rightfully deserve recognition.

It would be impossible not to highlight military heroes who put everything on the line for their respective countries. As an American, I beam with pride for the men and women in uniform.

The special forces are rightfully held in high regard by me as they have to tap into a mindset that few can achieve. It amazes me that they have such a degree of wherewithal to even get through training, much less deployment and mission execution.

In researching for this book, and to better understand how to embrace everything life throws our way, I began looking into other stories of overcoming adversities. The military has many examples of preparation, mission execution, adversity, and outcome.

The special forces, like the Navy Seals, go through very rigorous training. This training is to prepare them mentally, as much as anything else, for what they might face. To see people go through hell, and yet come out as inspirational lights of this world, is incredible.

A Shining Example of Moxie:

I want to highlight the story of Jason Redman. The man and his story embody Moxie:

Gut Punch

A "Life Ambush" as Jason Redman calls it in his book *Overcome,* is "a catastrophic series of events that knock the wind out of you, pin you to the pain and forever alter your reality." To date, my most extreme life ambush was my first born's cancer diagnosis.

The above definition of a "Life Ambush" fits to a "T" what happened to me. Redman states that most people will experience five life ambushes in a lifetime. Some we can see coming, while others will be a surprise attack with no way to be prepared.

The examples are broad from a medical diagnosis of self or a loved one, a break up, divorce, loss of a loved one, financial catastrophe, natural disaster, man-made disaster, tragedy, or, God forbid, the loss of a child.

These moments are universal experiences for us all, to varying degrees, nonetheless, they are a common thread in the existence of all mankind. The fact that we will all experience "Life Ambushes" is the primary reason to cultivate a Moxie Mindset.

In Jason Redman's work with Wounded Warriors, he has identified three groups of people and illustrates how they respond to life ambushes. They are as follows:

1. Victim - this group is consumed by the circumstance that happened to them. They become a victim and will succumb to the negativity associated with it.
2. Survivor - this group is simply survivors, and is the most common. They are focused on just getting through, and are pretty much stagnant in life; never becoming more.
3. Overcomer - they define themselves not by the challenge, but by their ability to overcome. They become stronger.

Athletes:

As a huge sports fan, especially football, and the Arkansas Razorbacks, I wanted to have a term that had a connection to us and our story.

Sports are controlled by adversity. In watching a game, challenges, strategy, skill, and beliefs are all on display. I think they are a great way to learn about human nature, and we can learn a great deal by understanding the psychology and mindset in sports, especially behind successful teams, players and coaches.

All of my life I've heard Moxie used as a way to positively describe a lot of quarterbacks, but it is not limited to them.

We draw a lot of inspiration from athletes as they are great examples of what it is to have Moxie.

SECTION 3

"The Blue Zone Protocol"
And
"Regenerative Health"
"Regenerative Agriculture"
"Regenerative Business"

Our experience with childhood cancer has been a rollercoaster, and very difficult. With that said, overall, Lander has done fantastically in comparison to what could have been our reality. Since he has done so well, I feel an obligation to share specifics of the lifestyle we implemented to help anyone else going through difficulties or, even better, help to avoid them altogether. Almost everything I say is anecdotal in Lander's particular case.

The research I'll bring together and share will prove the positive health impacts and I pray for assistance in overcoming the terrible affliction we know as cancer.

Looking back, I now have a better understanding of the benefits of many, the steps we took, and their positive impact.

The first thing we did was address Lander's diet, removing added sugars, processed foods - including flours, meats, and dairy. We focused on whole vegetables, avocados, mushrooms, nuts, and limited fruits.

The diet we implemented, which we refer to as *The LanderMan Plan*, has evolved considerably since the start, and will continue to grow. Most notable additions from the beginning were grass-fed meat, farm fresh eggs, wild-caught cold-water fish, butter, and ghee, along with animal proteins such as whey and collagen.

I've pulled a lot of the foundational principles we used for Lander from *Longevity Research.*

My thinking is, if we can understand what the most extended-living populations/communities are doing, we can learn to apply them to our lives.

My initial look into this work came from the research of Dan Buettner's, *The Blue Zones.* They are simply areas that Buettner, Gianni Pes, and Michel Poulain identified as places around the world where people live the longest. Buettner and his team literally draw a blue line around them, hence the name.

My home state of Arkansas is overall very unhealthy. It is a state that ranks in the bottom 3 in almost all health-related categories.

In all of the Blue Zones, modern chronic diseases are extremely rare or even nonexistent. If we are going to beat cancer, we need to understand the diet and lifestyle of those who don't have the disease. There is a stark contrast to the way Blue Zones live, and our modern-day life. Quite frankly, they don't have the same lifestyle, or eat the same way as we do.

While there are many centenarians (people living into their 100's), the modernization of certain Blue Zone communities is now causing a decreasing life expectancy for younger generations yet another statistic from which we can take into consideration.

If we can apply, and come together in creating a Blue Zone in Arkansas, we can do it anywhere in the world.

For instance, going back to Lander and the initial decisions we made around his diet, those choices remain remarkably similar to the principal characteristics of Blue Zone communities. From there, I wanted to learn which components had the most significant impact, and the reasons why. The two areas I focused on were Greece (Ikaria and Mount Athos) and Okinawa, Japan.

https://www.bluezones.com/exploration/ikaria-greece/

https://thefullnester.com/eat-like-a-monk-the-mount-athos-diet/

https://www.bluezones.com/exploration/okinawa-japan/

The reason I put so much faith into longevity is that there are proven long-standing track records. Lifestyle is a huge factor, and their steady diet is time-tested, unlike so many fad diets. In my view, there are numerous clearly evident credibilities.

I check any new information or recommendation I come across against longevity principles. It is essential to note, it's not only relevant to *what* they do, but maybe even more significant is *how* they do it. For this reason, I have a hard time getting behind the carnivore diet and I also check out soy and legume products very carefully with regards to how they are raised (organic, non-GMO) and processed for consumption (soaked, pressure cooked, or fermented).

I own a third-generation farmer's market-style grocery business, Me & McGee Market, in Arkansas that connects me directly to farmers, restaurants, food service, the healthcare industry, and consumers. Therefore, I have a front row into the food chain and operate a hub of sorts.

I see, and have seen, the interconnection between medicine, diet, agriculture and business. With that in mind, it seems non-productive and ineffective to be "warring factions" within that circle.

With that said, in focusing on creating healthy ecosystems in the human body, by combining a thriving environment with sound business practices, the result effectively creates the side effect of problem eradication.

It is my firm belief that in striving to create a Blue Zone in Arkansas, we can solve copious amounts of problems. Chronic diseases, including cancer, could disappear. Resilience in the environment and economy can increase, and life for everyone can be improved in both quality and quantity.

Arkansas a Future Bluezone Community?

Arkansas is my home. I was born and raised in the Arkansas River Valley which sits between the Ozark and Ouachita Mountains. The contours of the area are vast and it is known as The Natural State.

The beauty of my state lies in contrast to its unfortunate downside. Arkansas ranks close to the bottom (48th), when compared to other healthy lifestyle states. To further spotlight the adverse effects of unhealthy living, Arkansas sadly ranks high on the list for extremely poor health. Obesity, diabetes, cardiac disease and cancer are rampant.

I love my state and am passionate about strengthening its rural areas. Home to around three million people, commodity cropland is vast, and numerous cattle operations dot the countryside.

By applying the principles in this book, we can strive to improve the quality of life, take care of the environment, and create financial resilience.

Even before Lander's journey, I've been obsessed with the concept of prosperity. To me it's always been about living a high quality of life. Being prosperous. Early in life I simply focused on the financial aspects with a desire to be rich and teach others to be financially independent, even coining a blog "Sowing Prosperity".

Another way to put my audacious goal is to create a "Prosperity Zone".

Merriam Webster's definition of prosperity: *"Prosperity is the condition of being successful or thriving."*

As I've gotten older and experienced life it has become increasingly evident health, relationships, family and contribution are all parts of prosperity. I'm still as passionate about entrepreneurship and financial independence as I've ever been but now with the focus of those endeavors being on improving our world.

> *A healthy man wants a thousand things; a sick man only wants one.* - Confucius

In the context of a prosperous life, I will break down the areas of focus into three parts more connected than I ever realized.

Part 1.   Regenerative Health
Physical, mental, and emotional longevity

Part 2.   Regenerative Agriculture
(Regeniculture)
Agriculture with environmentally sound practices, leading to positives on all facets.

Part 3.   Regenerative Business
Entrepreneurship, Creation, Growth, and Financial Resilience

PART 1

Regenerative Health

I like to focus on the positive aspects of health. Some of the happiest and healthiest people have been studied through longevity.

A key point for longevity is that it is the opposite of chronic sickness. By embracing the positive, we can eliminate many of the horrors we face with poor health.

Heart disease, stroke, cancer, Alzheimer's, and diabetes are chronic killers increasing at a very alarming rate. Even with modern advancements in healthcare, it looks as if we are not winning the war. Cancer, in particular, is compounding at alarming rates and is becoming incredibly common in younger individuals.

Cancer is the primary focus in regard to health. Upon hearing my son's diagnosis, coupled with my extensive ensuing research, the world of the "Emperor of All Maladies" - the perfect disease, in many ways, was opened up to me.

From the beginning of my son's journey, I said, "God will do His part, the doctors will do theirs, and daddy will do his, to save and heal Lander."

From the get-go, I spent every waking moment researching to find solutions to give Lander every opportunity to beat cancer. I threw out all preconceived ideas, prejudices, and beliefs. I would look into any and everything that might help but wouldn't hurt my child.

I began to look into alternative cancer approaches, biohacking, longevity, ayurvedic medicine, and functional medicine. Researching alternative approaches to fighting cancer led me down many rabbit holes, but I was more often able to connect and apply something from everything.

Dave Asprey and Bulletproof Radio became the core of what I applied while going down different paths, always returning to regroup with some of his work before repeating the discovery cycle.

I believe I have every book Dave has written. His approach to cause and effect, results-based measurements of success, was a draw for me. His interviewing of experts has opened me up to information I may have never discovered.

All of this can also be said for Dr. Mark Hyman and his podcast Doctor's Farmacy. It's a wealth of knowledge, and I couldn't be more appreciative.

Lander went from stage 4 to cancer-free in 8 months. As of this writing, we are a year and a half old with no sign of disease.

My goal is to open up to ideas that could impact your life like Dave and Dr. Hyman have for me.

Regenerative Medicine including Functional Medicine looks at the root causes of disease. In almost all cases, the food we eat is the culprit.

When the diet is wrong, medicine is of no use. When diet is correct, medicine is of no need. Ayurvedic Proverb

Having lost my grandfather, Larry McGee, to cancer, along with my son's diagnosis of stage 4 kidney cancer, my theme for Lander's journey has always been, and I reiterate, "God will do His part, the doctors will do theirs, and I will do mine." Overcoming cancer and sharing resources is a passion that I work on daily in one form or another.

Blue Zones and Longevity

Our experience with childhood cancer has been a very difficult rollercoaster. With that said, overall, he has done superbly in comparison to what could have been our reality. Since he has done so well, I feel an obligation to share specifics of the lifestyle we implemented in hopes of helping anyone else going through difficulties, or even better, helping avoid them altogether. Most everything I say is anecdotal in Lander's particular case. In the research, I'll bring together and share that which will prove the positive health impacts and I pray for assistance in overcoming the terrible affliction we know as cancer.

What do Blue Zones have in common?

- When their stomachs are about 80 percent full, they stop eating. This helps reduce weight gain.
- They eat their smallest meal at dinnertime.
- Their diets are made up of mostly plants, beans, and they tend to avoid eating meat.
- The folks only eat about 3 to 4 ounces of meat about five times a month.
- Blue Zoners drink about 1-2 glasses of alcohol a day, and rarely exceed that amount.
- The communities are mostly free of heart disease, obesity, cancer and diabetes.
- The cultures value faith, family, and social gatherings.

The most intriguing part of longevity was the extremely low existence of chronic diseases. My thinking is if I can understand and apply what the people around the world without these problems are doing, I can improve Lander's life, as well as the rest of the family.

Diet is huge but the social and lifestyle components are essential.

This study led me to *The Longevity Diet* by Valter Longo and another look into the depths of the applicable practices that can be used to increase longevity.

Adding to my love for longevity and biohacking is *The Switch: Ignite Your Metabolism with Intermittent Fasting, Protein Cycling, and Keto* by James W. Clement. He is a lawyer and entrepreneur turned research scientist who has devoted the past two decades to understanding the science of life extension. He is best known for his *Supercentenarian Research Study,* which he started in 2010 with Professor George M. Church of Harvard Medical School.

Without being overly technical, autophagy is the process in which our bodies clean up cellular waste. The process is amplified during fasting and protein cycling due to mTOR. Cleaning up damaged and waste cells is exceedingly important in overcoming and preventing cancer.

Clement's work has been a major cohesive component to *The Landerman Plan,* in large part because of the ranged perspective and attention to cause and effect over a preconceived school of thought due to training. The scientific approach, in a holistic way, brings many of the specific areas of nutrition, biology, chemistry and general health together in a latticework of models.

In looking at dairy products through the understanding of many disciplines, such as Functional Medicine, Longevity Research, BioHacking, Ayurvedic, and even popular diets like Paleo, and Whole30, there is a lot of support for eliminating, or at a minimum, significantly reducing dairy.

When I refer to conventional or modern dairy, I mean commercial operations in which the animals are living an industrialized life. Not getting into the ethical argument, but they aren't living as cattle should, and the trade-off is negative.

I'm intrigued by the study of Longevity. "Blue Zones" is a name for areas with a high population percentage of individuals living to 100, coined by Dan Buettner. His book *Blue Zones* is a great read. Here are the studied locations: Okinawa, Japan; Sardinia, Italy; Nicoya, Costa Rica; Icaria, Greece; and among the Seventh-day Adventists in Loma Linda, California. It's a goal of mine to compile and relay information in a way that creates a Blue Zone of our own, even if not geographically.

Understanding why specific populations live longer gives insight into lifestyle choices to help us better import quality and length of life for ourselves. It is interesting to note, in these populations, there is a lack of the chronic diseases that plague the modern world, giving us another area of focus and better understanding. Longevity allows us to adapt to a preventative mindset. After personally watching so many loved ones and patients suffer when I was working EMS, I'm all for eliminating all preventable diseases and helping ease the lives of those that may be afflicted.

Noticeably lacking in Blue Zones is the consumption of dairy as we know it. The dairy they do consume is in a raw or unprocessed manner from sheep, goats, and A2 cattle breeds like Guernsey, Jersey, Charolais, and Limousin. Those breeds of cattle have a different protein make-up than the modern dairy cattle like Holstein. The science behind this is exciting, but the thing to take away is that our bodies process the milk of goats differently than the common breeds of cattle in modern dairy, making it easier for most to digest the milk from goats.

In *the Longevity Diet* by Valter Longo, Ph.D., his first principle is "Eat a mostly vegan diet with some fish." On the subject of dairy, he recommends refraining in almost all cases - another great book with a ton of useful information.

Interesting Analogy on the Human Body

In Valter Longo's book *The Longevity Diet*, he frames the human body as an army of cells always at war. The enemies Longo lists are oxygen and other DNA and cell-damaging molecules. Also, the immune system is continuously battling bacteria and viruses. Like the needs of an actual army of rations, ammunition, and other equipment, the body needs proteins, essential fatty acids, minerals, vitamins, and even sugars for battles within and outside cells. Insufficient amounts of nutrients lead to the body's inability to repair and replace, and slows down, or even stops, the defense system. Damage then accumulates, and harmful organisms like fungi and bacteria proliferate.

Without appropriate nutrients, essential bodily functions are unable to be performed at an optimal level, if even at all.

The most basic way to offset several deficiencies is by taking a high-quality multivitamin with minerals. An Australian study showed taking a multivitamin had a positive effect on a person's ability to deal with stress, and by impacting mood in individuals with poor nutrition.

I believe getting our nutrients from the food we eat is the best way, but it isn't always easy. A multivitamin is like added insurance. The caveat being low quality multivitamins are at best useless and at worst harmful. Understanding levels of minerals and fat-soluble vitamins is crucial to not overdo it. A health team is important to utilized supplements properly especially in conjunction with another supplementation.

Other vital components are the essential fatty acids, Omega 3 and 6, which are involved in critical processes like inflammation and blood clotting. Inflammation in bodily function is vital for health when speaking of proper immune function and the natural response to injury. However, chronic inflammation is credited with many of the health problems of today. Omega 6 fatty acids are pro-inflammatory, while omega 3 is anti-inflammatory. Unfortunately, the modern Western diet is very high in omega 6 and low in omega 3.

The importance of a much more balanced ratio has become a focal point for me due to the emphasis in longevity research. James Clements's work has shown a scary skew of Omega 6 in stark comparison to our Paleolithic-aged ancestors, who consumed closer to a ratio of 4 to 1. Most estimations I've seen start at around 16 to 1 going way higher in modern diets.

Omega 6 fatty acids are found in pretty much everything. Vegetable oils, like soybean, are very high in omega 6 as well as conventionally raised meat products. This is one of many reasons the LanderMan Plan lists them on the "avoid" list. So many of the experts claim excessive omega 6, especially in an oxidative form, leads to metabolic diseases such as cancer.

Walnuts, which are touted as high in as high omega 3, consist of almost five times omega 6; therefore, they don't need to be looked at to balance the ratio. Meat products, butter, and ghee from grass-fed animals and cold-water fish like salmon are the best way to get omega-three from dietary means.

Characteristic of Cancer:

Angiogenesis:
A common characteristic across almost all types of cancers is the forming of new blood vessels; a process known as angiogenesis, to support tumor growth. These additional blood vessels bring nutrients such as glucose and amino acids required by cancer cells. The vessels are spindly and threadlike, similar to varicose veins, but are sufficient to support and facilitate cancer cells to grow and spread. Malignancy is when a cancer cell breaks off and travels in the bloodstream to another part of the body, establishing another tumor.

Understanding this part of the cancer process is crucial to figuring out how to cure many forms. If we can stop the tumor from receiving the substances it needs to thrive, we can kill it and make other therapies more effective. This is one route by which we can take the fight against cancer.

A fantastic thing about this, is many plant compounds are known to be antiangiogenic, or they stop, or kill, the formation of new blood vessels.

Potent plant compounds can be found all over and can be utilized by eating them or taking them in supplement form.

Some Antiangiogenic Compounds – https://www.ncbi.nlm.nih.gov/pmc/articles/PMC1891166/

- Aloe Vera leaf and pulp extracts
- Artemisinin – Sweet Wormwood
- Curcumin – Turmeric
- Protocatechuic acid – Green Tea
- Flavonoids: apigenin, fisetin – German chamomile
- Omega-3 fatty acids (eicosapentaenoic acid, docosahexaenoic acid)
- Panax Ginseng (saponins: 20(R)- and 20(S)-ginsenoside-Rg3)
- Resveratrol – Grapes
- Quercetin – Capers, Onions
- Soy isoflavones (genistein, daidzein)
- Selenium
- Vitamin D

Another great resource is Dr. William Li https://drwilliamli.com/how-we-can-starve-cancer-with-food/

There are unlimited things we don't know about the benefits of different compounds, or have a full grasp of why they are vital to optimal health, with Antiangiogenic being but one.

Ways of getting health promoting compounds are diet, juicing, and supplements.

Some of the Cancer Specialists I've studied and are worth looking into:

- Otto Warburg
- Ralph Moss - Moss Reports
- Max Gerson
- Nicholas Gonzolas
- William Li

Diets:

I believe focusing on things within my control is the best use of my time and energy. This focus led me to see how vital a healthy diet can contribute to overall well-being. I've seen estimates of up to 35% of environmental causes of cancer are dietary related, with tobacco attributing up to 25%. I imagine that the number of dietary related cancers is higher. Regardless, diet is considerable, and avoiding harmful foods is essential.

There are layers to the diet, and there are a multitude of books on the topics. In my day today, I recommend three cookbooks to everyone because it's easy to get inundated with conflicting information. I also stress the cookbooks to most people because it's the book's consented version with actionable recipes.

1. *Bulletproof Diet Cookbook* - Dave Asprey
2. *Wahls Protocol Cookbook* - Dr. Terry Wahls
3. *Pegan Diet Cookbook* - Dr. Mark Hyman

These three cover almost everything you need to know. (Feel free to be like me and have 100's of books on nutrition and health but it's easy to get overwhelmed).

Part of Me & McGee Market is Lander's Corner, a health food store where we carry the products, including supplements, we use in our own lives.

I'm a huge proponent of supplements. Simultaneously, there is an industry of shady dealing and cons; when quality products are used, it's life-changing, with the quality of life improving.

Supplements have arguments on both sides. The primary fight against supplements I hear and agree with is - nutrients should be gotten from the food we eat. Yes, they should, but unfortunately, as we dive deeper and deeper, it will become clear that this is a nearly impossible goal to achieve.

However, with improved farming practices, the nutrient density of produce and meats will provide much of the needed compounds of health from food.

Common Deficiencies:

1. Gut Microbiome Diversity
2. Vitamins
3. Minerals
4. Omega 3's
5. Enzymes
6. Phytochemicals, Antioxidants, Plant-based compounds

I try to make things as simple as I can. Here is my oversimplification of disease as a whole. (Again, I'm not traditionally educated, just self-taught).

The two primary causes of disease are toxicity and deficiency. As such, they must be addressed for prevention and healing in any situation.

Toxicity:

Merriam Webster defines toxicity as: "the quality, state, or relative degree of being poisonous."

In our understanding, anything that causes harmful effects on the body is a toxin.

Common examples of toxins are heavy metals, mold, and pesticides. Toxins, that many people might not think about or disagree with, are high blood glucose levels found in pre-diabetic or diabetes. A medical example of a severe acute condition is diabetic ketoacidosis. This is a complication in which ketones increase to a poisonous level in the body.

I also include food allergies in the toxin topic. Many people have no idea they have issues with food because they affect everyone differently, manifesting in so many unexpected ways. For example, for a lot of people, gluten would be considered a toxin. Gluten is a protein found in grains, most commonly wheat.

There is a wide range of degrees of gluten issues from celiac being the most severe, to mild seasonal allergy-type symptoms. It is not uncommon for gluten-sensitive individuals to be tired, get headaches, depression, gas, diarrhea, bloating, cramps, and stomach pain. This will become more and more understood and accepted as time goes on. Not long ago, leaky gut syndrome was laughed at and called a quackery topic.

Gluten is a massive problem of which most people are completely unaware. For me specifically, if I eat anything with gluten I get extremely sick - from cramping, gas, and even diarrhea.

The main way I've found to avoid gluten is to completely remove it from our diets in the way of processed foods. There is no good reason to eat it. By doing this simple rule, it's easier to avoid the other health busters, vegetable oils and sugar.

Sourdough Bread:

I've found eating real sourdough bread causes none of the stomach issues from other gluten-containing foods. The long fermentation process breaks down the gluten and in most cases, does not cause problems. So it's not gluten-free but it is a gluten-friendly bread option. Studies have also shown real sourdough to have a lower glycemic index, meaning eating it won't spike blood sugar like other types of breads.

For a long time, I didn't think I liked sourdough. I've grown to love it and it is the only bread we eat. Any other bread causes extreme stomach pain, bloating and gas. It's eye opening just how bad gluten and processed foods are once you've' removed them for an extended time.

Easy Recipe

1. Sliced Sourdough toasted
2. Place sliver of Butter on hot toast
3. Drizzle yacon syrup (low glycemic sweetener with minerals and prebiotics) Favorite Brand is Z!nt (Not a typo)
4. Sprinkle with cinnamon

One of Lander's favorite snacks. I take this opportunity to give him greens drinks and supplements.

Deficiencies:

The other side of the health coin is a deficiency. The foundation is nutrition and the nutrients that should be gotten through our diets.

Here is an outline of some of the most well-known to show the significance of vitamins and mineral deficiencies.

- Calcium - Osteoporosis, Rickets
- Iodine - Goiter
- Selenium - Keshan disease
- Iron - Anemia
- Thiamine (Vitamin B1) - Beriberi
- Niacin (Vitamin B3) - Pellagra
- Vitamin C - Scurvy
- Vitamin D - Osteoporosis, Rickets
- Vitamin A - Night Blindness
- Vitamin K - Haemophilia

Deficiency comes in many forms without a clinical-named diagnosis. The immune system can't function properly without zinc, magnesium, vitamin c, and vitamin d, among many others that we don't even understand yet.

As I've gotten further and further into my research, a couple of things have become apparent. It is almost impossible to get all of the necessary nutrients from food alone. To begin with, the primary reason is that many of the fruits and vegetables are deficient. Over time, in storage and transit, nutrients become further degraded. By the time we get a tomato from the grocery store in our kitchen, the nutrient value is a fraction of a homegrown tomato from 50 years ago.

This is an extremely important topic to understand as we get much more in-depth in the Regenerative Agriculture in Part Two of this book. Soil health is as vital as the nutrient content of the foods that are grown in it.

This is an essential step in understanding how we have become such an unhealthy society. Not only do we not eat enough fresh plants we are overindulging in processed foods utterly devoid of nutrients for a healthy life.

The goal of this book is to hit on topics that may be off the radar. To go more in-depth on nutrition, I highly recommend Dr. Terry Walhs's work. She has done a fantastic job of outlining and giving practical ways of implementing her protocol.

Deficiencies in Omega 3 fatty acids are a considerable problem as well. The Omega 6 to Omega 3 ratio is essential to maintain at closer to 1 to 1 but in the modern diet, it is astronomically skewed towards Omega 6.

Combating Deficiencies:

In a perfect world, we would all have access to healthy sustenance by having nearby local farms, producing naturally grown produce, meats, eggs, and dairy like in the Blue Zones regions of the world.

It can be challenging to get the daily vegetables grown in biodynamic healthy soils, loaded with plant compounds like phytochemicals, antioxidants, chlorophyll, and enzymes. All of the meat would be raised on high-quality forage and supplemented with garden scraps or excess produce from an overabundance of harvest. This would lead to omega 3 rich meat and eggs containing essential micronutrients.

In practice, this can be difficult to accomplish. I own and operate a farmer's market, a food service, and farms, and understand the food systems intently, and am striving to make the best foods available to my family and customers. I endeavor to buy the bulk of the items from responsible farmers and markets.

Sowing Prosperity - Educational Content like Books, Videos and a Podcast:

Luke 11:9-10
And so I tell you, keep on asking, and you will receive what you ask for. Keep on seeking, and you will find. Keep on knocking, and the door will be opened to you. For everyone who asks, receives. Everyone who seeks, finds. And to everyone who knocks, the door will be opened.

I love how God clears the pathway and brings the knowledge right to you when you seek it in earnest. One of the avenues that has blessed me immensely is Sowing Prosperity. https://sowingprosperity.com

I have had the opportunity to be joined by some amazing people that are leading spokespersons in their fields of expertise.

I can't think of a better way to impart the knowledge they shared with me, than by interweaving transcripts of their time spent with me on my podcast within the pages of this book. What you can learn from them is immeasurable.

(The podcasts are shared in their raw, unfiltered form. I believe the best knowledge will be gained by getting to know these experts in their warm and natural personae, just as they delivered their information to me...)

Podcast Transcript Number Two: Adam Payne Founder, Inventor, CEO, and Josh Bellieu CPE, UltraBotanica

In the mission of constantly trying to learn new things to apply to life, I visited with Adam Payne and Josh Beluie of *UltraCur* to learn more about the science and impact of curcumin.

Logan: I'm here at Me and McGee Market. And with all the research I've done, turmeric and curcumin in particular have come highly recommended as something to incorporate into our diet and lives. With that, I came across *Ultracur*, and that is a business right out of Oklahoma City. We're going to visit with Josh and learn a lot more about what this could do for our health.

All right, Adam, Josh, thank you all so, so much for joining us today. Just to kind of set this up, the way I became enamored with turmeric and curcumin and the other components of that is through our cancer journey. So my little boy was diagnosed with cancer in 2019. I just really dove into what can I do to help him. And so turmeric was a big part of what I believe matters in health and tracking that down, came across y'all with your company. I love that you weren't very far from us, you just right over in Oklahoma. And so wanted to get you on and talk about the products you have, y'all's story and just let's meet the people behind an amazing product.

Josh: Got it. I come out of the pharmaceutical industry so you have to forgive me for that. I was working with some researchers at the University of Oklahoma and the Oklahoma Medical Research Foundation that were really into natural medicine. And it's rare actually for hardcore, heavy duty, National Institute of Health funded researchers to have anything to do with natural medicine, because there's almost no funding for it. The funding is for the molecular mechanisms and all that stuff. But there were some researchers that were looking at turmeric and curcumin at the Oklahoma Medical Research Foundation, and they had a simple idea. The idea was that curcumin in its extracted form turns into an aggregate, a crystal. And all of the people that were trying to help curcumin get absorbed into the body because of all of the research around cancer and inflammation, because there's a lot of it over 18,000 published articles about cancer and inflammation just around the turmeric and curcumin.

But the problem with the curcumin is that when it's extracted and even in the turmeric group, it's a crystal. It's an insoluble crystal, that's like quartz crystals, right? So imagine trying to take a bunch of quartz crystals into your body and hoping that you would solubilize some of the silicone that's in the quartz and get it absorbed into your system. It just doesn't happen. You have to take massive amounts of curcumin for it to absorb in the body. So all of the pharmaceutical researchers like myself out there, they put on their little formulation hats and said, "Well, if we're going to try to improve the absorption of curcumin, we just need to make the crystal smaller, make nanoparticles of the curcumin. "When you make it something smaller, you exponentially increase the surface area. When you increase the surface area, you create more solubilization. So that's what everybody else was doing, except for these guys at the Oklahoma Medical Research Foundation. They said, "Look, screw that." That's a technical term.

Logan: That's a technical?

Josh: You have to use a screwdriver to do that.

"Screw that, we are going to drive the curcumin into a liquid matrix," which is a fancy way of saying, "We're just going to put it into solution." And so when it's in solution, you have single molecules of the curcumin and those single molecules of the curcumin are what our bodies need and what cancer needs, what our inflammation needs in order for it to make a difference. So we made this stuff, we sat around the table, in fact.

Liquid tincture around here, somewhere?

This is actually some of the original stuff.

Logan: Nice, nice.

Josh: From seven years ago.

So can you imagine guys sitting around the table doing shots of the liquid curcumin here, looking at each other, going, [crosstalk 00:04:40].

So here's one on that. And so this is still in solution and it's still viable. This was liquid curcumin that we made over six years ago. And to the horror of the scientists, they were horrified.

Logan: I know.

Josh: They really were. We made some of the stuff. We got some shot glasses and, a couple of us, we tried it. And the most astonishing thing about this is that, within two to three minutes, we had this buzzing feeling in our heads. We call it the Curcumin Buzz. And what was astonishing to me was that, I knew at that moment that not only was, it was those molecules of curcumin getting into my body, but for me to be feeling something in my head, meant that it was getting into my brain. So those molecules of curcumin [crosstalk 00:05:30] going through my gut, circulating it through my body, getting into my brain and we were feeling it.

And it was that turned on a switch inside my head and said, "There's something different about what we're doing here." And as simple as that sounds, just creating a liquid curcumin that drove us into a whole, another realm of research. And what that led us into was that we were able to develop something called liquid protein scaffold technology. We learned that curcumin, this is the simple insight that's patented right now is that curcumin would bind to protein before it would bind to itself. And so we present liquid curcumin to a protein scaffold.

So the molecules of curcumin bind to this protein scaffold, and as the body's digesting the protein, the curcumin has readily absorbed. Some people ask why don't we sell this stuff to people. And we used to, but you have to take a 12-ounce bottle of the liquid curcumin to get the same dose that you're getting in one of our capsules. So the liquid protein scaffold *UltraCur* technology is literally molecules of curcumin bound to this protein scaffolding.

Logan: All right. So to just kind of regroup on what, what we're talking about, we've known for 1000s of years through ayurvedic medicine, or whatever, that turmeric kind of Indian, Asian cuisines that use that, they don't have a lot of the diseases that we know, that's how they treat a lot of it. So umpteen scientific studies, turmeric, curcumin, they are improved of health. The problem, our bodies can't absorb hardly any of it. So I think one of the last-

Josh: Except, in traditional Indian cuisine, what do they do with the turmeric? [crosstalk 00:07:28] They cook, they cook it in oil, and that releases the molecules of the turmeric into the oil. So that yellow color is the molecules of the curcumin. And so they're getting some absorption there, but even with that, one capsule of our product is equal to over 100 grams of turmeric root [crosstalk 00:07:54] in terms of how much, how much material you're getting into the body. So you need a lot of turmeric. You would need to eat a lot of turmeric on a daily basis.

Logan: Yeah. Imagine just having a plate piled up to about here, and then sticking a spoon in it and eating that. [crosstalk 00:08:08].

Josh: Well, you would have to cook it, but eating the powder, you'd have a half a kilo of powder in order to get the same, what you would absorb with one of our capsules. Or you'd have to cook it, which is very too intense for most people in order to release the molecules out of the turmeric group into a molecular form.

Logan: That's what makes y'all's product so intriguing. And I think kind of why it works so well. So since I have been having y'all's product at the market, I've been giving out those little packets that you sent, the little samples. 100% of people have said that they have helped. So my mom, grandma, friends, we've got lady that helps us, she's family, more like an aunt, a lot of being prescribed gabapentin for neuropathy and other nerve pains. And they're absolutely loving.

Logan: Hold on one second. Boys?

Uh oh. We talked to a pharmaceutical guy, but Josh tell us a little bit about you while-

Josh: And I do want to mention too that Adam is the one that actually originally educated me on these population studies that they did. These are like global studies where they look at populations and they dial in to understand why in the world of the individuals in this area of the world, or this area of the world, not having high incidence of Alzheimer's, of cancers, of diabetes, and things like that. And they did one of these studies, what several decades ago, '50s and '60s. I mean, it was the '60s and '70s.

I mean, it was the epidemiologist, the statisticians that study populations that really discovered that turmeric was responsible for lower Alzheimer's rates, lower cancer rates and lower diabetes rates. Because when they looked at all these populations, there were certain populations that just had lower cancer rates, lower diabetes, and Alzheimer's, and the only factor that was present in those populations was if turmeric was a daily part of their diet. If they weren't taking three to four grams of turmeric into their daily dietary intake, then you have these lower diseases and everywhere else, it was hard. So, that started the whole craze. That's why there's 19,000 plus published articles about turmeric.

And as Adam will tell you, when they dialed into the turmeric root, it's a rhizome, really only about 3% of that is what they call curcuminoids. And there's actually, I think about five of them, Adam?

Adam: Three.

Josh: Three? Okay. Three of them. And those that's only 3% of turmeric, but they found that to be the active agent that was responsible for these unique changes in people's bodies and health. And so enter Adam and his guys, and well actually Adam and me, I have a dear friend that I've been in business with for a number of years. Adam and I occasionally would attend the morning men's group, prayer, hanging out, talking men together. And I had kept missing him, he'd been there when I wasn't there, I'd been there.

And my friend goes, "Josh, I met this guy the other morning and they're doing some really interesting things out at Oklahoma Medical Research Foundation. They're working actually with curcumin," which my radar went up because I've been into alternative health since I was 16. I'm 61 now. And I got interested, but he said, "But he was talking about how individuals that are dealing with pain, which finds its root in inflammation and unhealthy inflammatory response in the body that that is what's triggering the pain." And as they begin to give this invention, this technology that Adam invented, because Adam is the guy that had the idea, how do we take this liquid, which is hard to ship around, and it tastes yucky and people don't want to chug a bunch of it every day. And so he's the one that had that interesting God drop when he was dropping the material on his finger and watching it bind to proteins in his skin.

And you drop this liquid on your finger, seven days later, even with bleach wipe, you're going to have a little bit of yellow stain there because it just instantly has this affinity. That's one of the patents that they filed and received. So I thought I've got to meet this guy. I will rewind the tape a little bit for me. I had the pleasure of being a part of a two-man startup. And our primary product was a product that people would use to relieve pain that was applied topically, a variety of different natural ingredients. We had a dear friend of ours that made it here right here in Oklahoma. We ended up with well over a million active customers that were blown away by our product. But during that period of time, I got to learn what pain does to marriages. What pain does to a person's ability to work, what it does for their ability to relate to their children or their grandkids, their spouses, their brothers, sisters.

Pain just takes everything down to this horrible, common denominator, and it debilitates people. And it changes the way they even think about lives. Adam knows because he struggles with something that even our curcumin doesn't help. It's a difficult thing that he's going through. But when I went and met with Adam and we got to talking and I knew about curcumin, but I didn't know that it was... I mean, I've been seeing it everywhere, but all of a sudden, we're faced with the idea of, "Wow." Adam has this material. He's been giving away in capsule form to friends. And oftentimes the very next morning, they're calling him. And of course, he's got a pharmaceutical background and it's like, "Adam, you didn't give me a drug. Did you?"

He was like, "Why?" And it's like, "Because I got out, worked in my garden yesterday for five hours, moved things around, raked leaves, hadn't done that in years and I didn't pay any price. And I woke up this morning without any stiffness." Now this is just shocking news. When I began to hear these stories, I'm like, "I have to meet this guy." So we get together and we're talking. And as he's educating me about curcumin, I realize, "Oh my goodness, how in the world do you separate yourself as you're bringing this unique invention to market that can change people's lives in such a short time? How do we distinguish ourselves from the others out there?" Well, we came up with the idea, "Hey, wait a minute." I did a little discovery interview with Adam. And I found out that people taking the original *Ultracur* product, the orange lid, I think that's probably sitting on a shelf back there. If they would take two capsules twice a day, they would experience a transformational result if they had been dealing with discomfort, stiffness, pain.

And so, we've done a huge sampling program at my previous company. And it had been so successful to differentiate us from other topical pain relievers out there. So we came up with the idea, made up these cool little envelopes, sealed them up. And I said, "I know what I'm going to do, Adam, I'm going to go out to compounding pharmacists, master herbalists, licensed clinical nutritionists, MDs, osteopaths, integrative and functional medicine specialists, nurse practitioners. And I'm going to drop off enough product to them to give to five of their patients. And I'm going to tell them, 'Don't give this to anyone that has occasional pain. Give this to individuals that are dealing with daily, chronic pain.

And from my standpoint, the worst, the better, we really want to see how this works. Will you participate in this with us?"

And so I went and I told them, "I won't leave you this free product, unless you will promise me to test them in five of your patients or customers." We went to a few independent health food stores as well. I had people calling me, Logan, for orders five days after that, because they began to give it to coworkers that were in pain, give it to their spouse, give it to their grandpa, their mom, their dad, and immediate results were taking place for individuals. And so that's what became our mantra for distinguishing ourselves from the other products out there is, don't believe us, try it and see for yourself if results are going to happen in a short window. And my personal story is kind of interesting because when Adam and I first met, I said nothing to him about the fact, you can kind of see I'm slender try to take care of myself.

Don't drink soda, pop, eat a real clean diet, take a lot of supplements. I'd been experiencing five years of inflammation that was manifesting and some pretty intense pain in my hips. Even sitting in a cushion chair like this for about five minutes. If I was doing this interview back then I would have gotten up and started to stretch. Car trips were just an abomination. They really, really hurt. So when we were leaving our first meeting, he was like, "Hey, you want to take a bottle with you?" And I said, "Sure." And I thought, "I'm going to kick the tires on this stuff and see if these stories are true." I started taking it. Now I'm an outlier. It took me five days, but I think he and I met on a Tuesday. And by a Saturday I was basically pain-free in my hips and was completely shocked.

Couldn't even in my mind reconcile, why is this happening? How did this work like that? It's not a drug. I don't have any side effects, unwanted side effects in any way. The end of that story though, is I used to ride motorcycles a lot and do stupid things in cars when I was a teenager. I did, and I wrecked a few times. And so I had had a shoulder that for about 17 years, I had been told by doctors, "Let me give you steroids shots," which I didn't want and didn't take. And they said, "Your only other alternative is rotator cuff surgery. Wasn't going to let anybody cut on me, Logan and I had lost. I used to love working out with weights. I had lost so much strength in this one, probably about 40 to 50%. And it was one of those weird things where I love to sleep on my right side.

Couldn't sleep on my right side, only intermittently over the 17-year period of time. If I moved really quick to grab something that fell or something, it's like, you're going to pay a horrible price. Couldn't reach over the back seat to pick up my briefcase out of the back. I'd have to get out of the car.

Logan: We get it. We get it.

Josh: Two weeks later, I was experiencing no popping in my shoulder. It was so strange. And then I began to kind of test the waters and basically, I'm about 95% strength back in this. I can reach out and pick up 40 pounds now, throw a stack of garbage or leaves into something with one arm. I could not do that. And so, I had this profound experience with it. And fortunately, our individuals out in the field that began to get this product just began to give it away to their customers.

Adam: They experienced the same thing.

... and they literally a lean startup company. Didn't have a lot of money for advertising, really no money for advertising, all of a sudden organically. And then doctors get interested. Adam met a doctor on an airplane, beautiful guy from here in Oklahoma City. He went to an international symposium of all these doctors in Germany, about 200 people from about 40 different countries. And he said, "Adam, can I talk about your stuff? I'm that impressed with it." And from there, it just kind of began to grow and blossom for us. It's remarkable.

I know from our limited experience, because honestly, we haven't had it very long here at the market, but it is verbatim what y'all are saying, it has been our experience. I wanted to hit on another thing real quick.

So the kind of the standard treatment for pain is NSAIDs and opioids, right? And so what I am so excited about is,

Logan: And steroids.

Adam: is, and steroids, an option for people to at least check out to say, "Hey, these..." Because we know the there's negatives from mitochondrial dysfunction with NSAIDs, the opioid dependency, constipation, blah, blah, blah, blah. So the side effects scare me for as a parent, as a son to see my family go through it. So to have an option that they're saying, "Hey, I'm not having the pain and I'm not needing these other things," is a big, big deal for me.

So curcumin works in a very different mechanism from anything else. It's called, the scientific term is Pleiotropic. It means it interacts with a whole bunch of things, but if you can get it in a molecular form and you can get it into your body, then it will interact with something inside the cells called the NF-kappa beta site inside the cells. And that is the mechanism by which that's the throttle. It's like the gas pedal inside yourself. The gas pedal tells the cell how inflamed it is or how much inflammation is going on around it. So when you have inflammation that is not healthy, out of balance, like from arthritis, like from a sports injury, it will actually shift the cell from unhealthy inflammation to a healthy inflammation. We call it a Th1 to Th2 response. The Th1 is the attack, right? And I'll give an example. Let's say we've all been hit in the head with a baseball bat or a ball or something like that. What happens?

Logan: A goose egg.

Adam: A goose egg. You know what's inside that goose egg is not filled with liquid. That goose egg is filled with millions and millions of immune cells that have rushed into that area, looking for a fight. In fact, if you look at the capillaries, they express these little Velcro adhesion molecules, and when the immune cells that are just naturally in circulation, our body see that Velcro, they roll through the capillaries and into that space, isn't that amazing? So really what's happening, that's that is a perfect example of the immune response. The body is saying there's damage here. The cells scream out their 911 call, "We're hurt." And then the immune system sends in the first responders.

What happens in inflammation, in our joints, in our tissues when we're hurting is the body is doing the same immune response. It's sending in immune cells, looking for a fight. Curcumin throttles back that signal. It tells the cells stop sending for the Calvary. Let's start to rebuild the tissue. And so it reestablishes homeostasis in, in our, in our joints, in our tissues, we call it helping our bodies achieve healthy inflammation or a healthy homeostasis. And so when you get curcumin into there, it's not specifically targeting the Cox1 or the Cox2, it's not a steroid telling your body to go into overdrive and cause you're in a fight or flight situation in the tissues. It's not a drug telling you to ignore the pain, which just causes more damage, right. It's actually going in there and helping you yourselves achieve a healthy status in terms of their inflammation response. The key is getting it in.

Josh: Yeah. So, Logan we've had the privilege because Adam being a researcher and then that beautiful event that took place when Dr. Brian Frank who's on our medical advisory board, went to Germany and spoke with these doctors. And Adam had the privilege of getting over there in one year as well. We have this network of opinion leaders and even key opinion leaders in the integrative and functional medicine space. And as we've done radio interviews with a number of these people, one of the favorite questions that I love to ask is, "Okay, you doctors that we're speaking with right now, in your opinion, how much of the disease that we suffer with worldwide is tied to what Adam was just talking about." This unhealthy inflammatory response that people are stuck in.

And he'll even tell you in a little bit about subclinical inflammation and what that means. The answers have astonished Adam and I both because our own medical advisory board, Dr. Brian, Frank instantly said 92% sitting next to him was a guy named who's a brilliant eye surgeon, American fellow college nutrition, key opinion leader, and then a consultant to many of the big pharmaceutical companies out there. He didn't blink an eye and said, Josh, in my humble opinion, at least 99%.

I don't agree with him. But it's everywhere. Inflammation is the primary driver for most human disease, cardiovascular disease, kidney disease, Alzheimer's, most of the human of the human diseases that people deal with have an inflammation component to it. I'll give an example. Cardiovascular disease is when plaque builds up inside our arteries inner veins, right? That plaque buildup is an inflammation response. The body is essentially, there's an inflammation going on in the wall of the artery. The artery protects itself by creating a plaque shield there as the immune cells embed inside of that artery wall. And that it creates a bony surface to protect itself. So to keep the circulation open so that... And that, we call it subclinical inflammation. That's subclinical inflammatory response because of our wonderful American diet, because of the damage that we caused to our bodies. And because we don't take care of ourselves, that those plaques build up over time.

What we learned also, because I studied Rheumatoid Arthritis for a long time, is that inflammation in our joints and in different tissues, inflammation in those tissues will actually leak over into our circulation. So if you have Rheumatoid Arthritis or if you have Sjogren's or Lupus or Psoriatic Arthritis, that inflammatory signal actually leaks out of those tissues and gets into our circulation causing inflammation everywhere. That's why people with rheumatoid arthritis have a lifespan that's seven to 10 years shorter than other people it's because of the cardiovascular risk and the brain risk and all these other tissues. It's crazy.

Logan: I think you hit on such an important point that it is such a wide range. It is lifestyle, it's diet, it's a lack or maybe too much exercise. It's the not having the micronutrients or other supplements that you really can't get unless you take a supplement. So just bringing awareness by having these type of interviews, being able to deal with the specialists, the experts in any given field. So, I mean, y'all are one of a wide range that I do is so important because I feel people need to be able to make their own decisions on how they want to deal with their life or whatever effects that they have and how to get over them. So guys, thank you y'all so much for taking the time. I am an absolute believer in the product. I'm excited that our paths have crossed and I fully anticipate visiting with y'all again.

Adam: So I have a recommendation for your listeners here. So if they're just looking for subclinical inflammation, healthy benefit, they feel good. One capsule of *UltraCur* twice a day will do wonders for blood chemistry and subclinical inflammation. And if people want to try the product, I know you have free samples. You have two capsules, twice a day of our original formula. Within two to three days, most people will either have a dramatic experience or it won't help. It's really true enough.

Josh: I can't emphasize enough, Adam just now like sucked my thoughts out of my brain for our parting thought, because so much of the time when people are taking our product, Logan, they have come because they'd had another powerful recommendation from a friend or loved one they trust that has said, "You guys relieved my pain," but I really want to tag into Adam's talk there. Do you want a better quality of life? Would you like to potentially avoid some of these devastating diseases that happen as we age? Gosh, I don't believe that there is a supplement out there.

There is a magic bullet or a panacea, but in my... Gosh, what now, it's been 36, 38 years of being in this arena and loving these kinds of things? This has come the closest to me for something that will affect liver enzyme levels, it will affect the oxidative stress in the heart. It will affect the overall inflammatory markers in the body. Your listeners, I would challenge them to get on pubmed.gov, P-U-B, M-E-D.gov, and type in curcumin in any disease. And it's probably been studying and they'll find out it's amazing, but then they'll find out if you don't get that curcumin in the bloodstream in a molecular form, that attaches to the cell receptor, you're not going to see these kinds of results.

Logan: Right. Thank you y'all.

Josh: Thanks, Logan. Appreciate you.

Logan: I'll visit with y'all soon and we'll keep spreading the good news.

Josh: We look forward to it. Thanks.

Cancer Stem Cells

I have a goal of a future without cancer. Effective treatments that are not worse than death. We envision a future with grandparents having more time to spend with family, and a future where parents are not taken too soon. Our hope is also for a future where children never have to know the ultimate fight. In essence, a cancer-free world.

My first personal experience with cancer was my grandfather, Larry McGee, diagnosed with non-Hodgkins lymphoma. He had a very long and difficult battle with many ups and downs. It is the rollercoaster that many know much too well.

Even dealing with my grandfather's battle, I was by no means prepared when I was told my little boy had Stage 4 cancer, in which he received conventional treatments of surgery, radiation, and chemotherapy as well as many other complimentary things.

Being nominated for The Leukemia and Lymphoma Society (LLS) 2021 Man of the Year was an incredible honor and has been a way to tie together many mutually beneficial aspects of my life.

While Lander is cancer-free, he must continue to undergo scans to monitor for relapse. I will cover much more in-depth as to why some specialists believe relapse is so common. Additionally, there are numerous negative effects of treatments, and rebuilding his little body is a long-term mission. I research every day as to how to overcome and prevent cancer. God allowed us to experience difficulties in which to grow and help others.

Lymphoma and leukemia are prevalent words that strike fear into our hearts. Leukemia is the most common childhood cancer. During our weekly visits and hospital admission to the Children's Oncology unit, I was exposed to many others in similar situations while getting to know the families and kids in their fights.

Those suffering from leukemia have abnormally high numbers of immature, dysfunctional white blood cells that crowd out the bone marrow interfering with the body's ability to create healthy blood cells.

Cure rates for leukemia are much better than they were even a short time ago. Estimates are upwards of 80% for most types. There are rare forms of the disease that initially go into remission, but then have a fatal relapse.

The visions we have of cancer-stricken individuals tend to be bald people with pale, grayish skin. They are most often weak and frail.

Another sad fallout from cancer is the effect it has on the families and caregivers. They are normally heartbroken and exhausted.

I often felt guilty when we had good news, because I watched so many babies struggle and eventually lose their lives. The unfairness was so unbearable.

However, the hard times motivated me to push through to find more effective and less harsh treatments.

There have been unbelievable movements forward, yet we are so far behind in implementing them. I truly believe we have overspecialized to the extent that we are losing cross-disciplinary movements. For that reason, I always find myself going back to integrative and functional medicine.

My goal is to bring all practices together to get better results, not divide or diminish any of the battlefronts. When we look at cancer statistics, we aren't winning the battle and maybe we should reframe the way we look at cancer. Declaring war on things doesn't mean casualty-free victory. Just one hundred years ago, the occurrence was around 1 in 100; today, it's close to 1 in 3. What has happened for such an abysmal progression? I believe our food is a massive part of the puzzle. Smoking and alcohol are prominent contributors. However, the way our food is processed, grown, and chemical exposures are areas where we can and should focus.

An eye-opening topic in cancer is cancer stem cells or CSC's.

There is debate regarding this topic but here is my summary. All cancer starts in stem cells through damage to mitochondria. As cancer develops, some of the daughter stem cells differentiate into non-stem cells. Cancer stem cells are the cancer cells that have not differentiated, yet are still stem cells which can replicate. Differentiated cells can no longer divide so although they are part of the tumor, they can't add to the tumor mass. They can't spread cancer if they break away from the tumor and travel to other areas of the body.

"Some say they're the cells from which a tumor originates," says Carla Kim, PhD, who researches lung stem cells in the [Children's Hospital Boston] Program. "Others think they're specialized cells within a tumor that help maintain it." [2]

CSC's and Cancer Therapy Resistance

"CSC's can generate a tumor when transplanted into an immune-deficient animal. Most CSCs are believed to be resistant to chemo- and/

or radiation- therapy, indicating the important roles CSCs play in cancer relapse and metastasis." [1]

It has been explained to me by an alternative cancer specialist that when looking at scans and seeing a reduction in the size of a tumor - the cells that are being destroyed are not cancer stem cells, but cancer differentiated cancer cells.

I'm not trying to scare people, but I believe this is extremely important. While treatment may appear to be working because tumors are getting smaller, the treatment may not be useful if the Cancer Stem Cells are not destroyed. This is where you hear of relapse after clear scans. It is because there are still CSC's in the body, and they are more aggressive and harder to kill.

"We're incredibly good at shrinking tumors, and incredibly bad at curing them," says Richard White, MD, PhD, an oncologist and clinical fellow in the Stem Cell Program at Children's Hospital Boston. [2]

Scott Armstrong, MD, Ph.D., a pediatric oncologist at Children's and the Dana-Farber Cancer Institute and affiliate member of the Stem Cell Program at Children's, likens cancer stem cells to queen bees: A hive collapses only if the queen is destroyed; if she isn't, the colony re-forms. White makes another analogy. "If you want to get rid of a tree, you could cut off the branches and hope it dies, but usually won't," he says. "Or you could cut out the root, which will kill the tree. Current chemotherapy removes the branches, not the root." [2]

All is not lost, far from it, but understanding this is vital. As I've covered in a previous https://meandmcgeemarket.com/food-as-medicine-radishes-juicing-and-angiogenesis/ post on angiogenesis, the characteristics of cancer and attacking them on all fronts, is part of the ability to overcome.

I can't stress this enough: any person with cancer needs an experienced and cohesive team made up of oncologists, integrative health care practitioners, spiritual and emotional mentors and cancer coaches.

My guiding principle is "God will do his part, the doctors/team will do theirs and I will do mine."

Plant-based compounds have been shown over and over to be used in pharmaceuticals. For example, Vincristine is a chemotherapy drug that Lander was given. The active ingredient is vinca alkaloids isolated from the rosy periwinkle, Catharanthus roseus. This plant has been traditional Chinese and Ayurvedic medicine, and now is a standard cancer therapy that has been around for over 50 years. Cancers treated with Vincristine include acute leukemia, Hodgkin's and non- Hodgkin's lymphoma, neuroblastoma, rhabdomyosarcoma, Ewing's sarcoma, Wilms' tumor (Lander's Diagnosis), multiple myeloma, chronic leukemias, thyroid cancer, and brain tumors.

I'm not saying eating rosy periwinkle will treat cancer. My point is plant-based compounds used with the direction of a healthcare professional can be a significant part of beating and/or slowing the disease.

An oncologist isn't going to recommend supplements or a diet. I pray I'm able to influence change in this area in the future. Looking at the factual data from reputable studies shows the statement I hear daily, "My oncologist said there is no proof XYZ, diet or nutrition affect beating cancer." There is a lot of proof and I provide links in all of my articles.

If your oncologist isn't supportive of you doing everything possible to save your own life, find a new one. There are plenty of outstanding doctors, oncologists, and specialists willing to be team members and not play God.

The reason a team is a must, especially with the inclusion of supplementation, is the following natural compounds have been shown to kill cancer stem cells. No one team member is going to have all of the answers yet can have the best answers for their given specialty.

Natural products and where they are found in which target cancer stem cells [4]

- Resveratrol - Grape Skin
- Curcumin - Turmeric
- Quercetin - A lot of plants - Dark Berries, Onions, Apples
- Piperine - Black Pepper
- Capsaicin - Pepper - Gives the Heat
- Berberine - A lot of plants, including Goldenseal
- Brefeldin A - Penicillin Fungus

Immunotherapy is also an area of excitement and showing promise in killing cancer stem cells. [3] Using the body's own immune system to attack and kill the cancer is another tool that may lead to more effective treatments.

Lander was a trooper during his journey, but we can learn every day while trying to bring together more effective ways to treat cancer.

I am not a medical specialist and do not give medical advice but I will create awareness and point those in need in the direction I would go in their situation. Again, a team of professionals is a vital part of the journey.

Footnotes

Cancer Stem Cells
[1] https://www.ncbi.nlm.nih.gov/pmc/articles/PMC3496019/
[2] http://stemcell.childrenshospital.org/treating-patients/
     probing-the-deadly-ways-of-cancer-stem-cells/
[3] https://www.ncbi.nlm.nih.gov/pmc/articles/PMC6468501/
[4] https://www.ncbi.nlm.nih.gov/pmc/articles/PMC5523038/

I've been very open with our cancer journey and for that reason many people come to me and ask for my advice. While I can't give medical advice, I tend to point them in the direction of a functional medicine doctor or research literature.

The most common issues I hear about are:
- Stomach Issues - Constipation, Diarrhea, Bloating, Cramping
- Headaches
- Pain
- Fatigue
- Poor Sleep

Common Diagnoses of Visitors or their Family Members
- Obesity
- Diabetes
- Cancer
- High Blood Pressure
- Alzheimers/Dementia
- Psychological

For myself and my family this is basically a list of the things I've found in researching how to help Lander have changed our lives.

What is the Human Microbiome

In the grand scheme of things, the human microbiome is a relatively new field of sturdy and refers to the microbial communities like bacteria, fungus and viruses that live in and on the human body.

Dr. Stephen Gundry's, The Plant Paradox got me focused on the "bugs" that live in our digestive tract. The impact, both positive and negative, from the organisms living in us is fascinating.

With the rise in gastrointestinal issues such as Celiac, IBS, Leaky Gut, Gluten Intolerance and Sensitivity, the microbiome is proving to be a significant factor. We have decimated our gut flora over the years by consuming pharmaceutical antibiotics and pesticides, of which many act as antibiotics. Additionally, through the modern diet, we are feeding the "bad bugs," as we call it at home.

This is a huge deal and must be at the core of what we do. The exciting part is how much we can help and positively impact our lives.

If you want to take a deep dive into gut health, I highly recommend the book *Total Gut Balance* by Mahmoud Ghannoum and Eve Adamson.

It helps me to think of our digestive tract as a jungle river valley. In its perfect form, it is a slow-moving, steady river with an incredibly diverse group of plants and animals living together. This river, made up of the small and large intestine, is about 28 feet long, and the jungle is home to an over 100 trillion bacteria jungle, weighing more than a few pounds with most living in the large intestine. When everything is balanced, all is well. Estimates indicate that 80% of our immune systems are in our gut. We are making the microbiome a considerable focus in *The LanderMan Plan*.

For our broad comparison, the animals and plants in the jungle are bacteria and fungi. The nutrients for a jungle are sunlight, air and water, and the food and water we drink. These nutrients are transported to and through the river to the ocean, also known as a toilet.

In the healthy way of life, there is a cycle of sunlight, air and water, used by a plant to grow. Periodically, parts of the plant die (like leaves or branches), creating organic matter such as leaves to feed other organisms. Animals eat parts of the plant - picture a rabbit eating grass, or an elephant eating leaves - keeping the plants from overgrowing, the rabbit runs around pooping, putting more nutrients in the ground. Just like a rabbit providing additional nutrients, bacteria in our gut break down things we eat, to be used by the body (like vitamins and antioxidants). The rabbit, getting eaten by larger animals, keeps their balance in check. This is the jungle lifecycle in a nutshell. Everything is interconnected.

If things get out of balance, problems arise. Say, for instance, the sun shines too much or not enough, the river floods or runs dry, the air or water becomes polluted - the jungle ecosystem suffers damage.

Let's look at an example: there is an explosion in the population of an invasive carnivorous predator. With a small population, the invader isn't causing issues but is now wreaking havoc on the community of other living creatures. The rabbits are completely eradicated, which in turn among other problems, leads to an overgrowth of plants. We would call this an infection in the human body, whether it's from a bacteria like H Pylori or yeast-like Candida. The medical approach to this is to kill the overpopulated invader by taking antibiotics. The thing about antibiotics or antifungals is that they don't discriminate, so it's a lot like spraying poison on the entire jungle to target the problem.

Now we have killed many of the beneficial plants and animals in the jungle, but still weren't able to kill the invader, so we respray the entire jungle again. Unfortunately, this time it's a more potent poison, destroying more and more of the useful living organisms and plants. This cycle is repeated over and over until the jungle looks nothing like its former self.

Chemotherapy, pesticides, alcohol, many medications, toxins, lack of sleep, stress, and even over sterilization all poison our jungle.

To save the jungle, we must stop applying the poison, reseed the plants, introduce native and beneficial animals, and give them the nourishment they need to thrive.

The good bugs do a host of crucial functions within the body. They play a role in the digestion, detoxification, and synthesis of many vitamins.

It's interesting that certain chemo drugs like cisplatin rely on gut microbes in destroying tumor masses.

Another critical component of the microbiome jungle is biofilms. Given the conditions in the gut are right, the body works to form a biofilm that acts as a barrier against bad guys. But when the conditions are adverse, the build-ups can be extremely problematic. A biofilm we are all familiar with is on your teeth in the morning. This is akin to bringing large amounts of landfill waste, mixing it with wet concrete, and dumping it all over. These form structures that are hard and detrimental to the ecosystem. They harbor Candida and are very difficult to manage.

We are in control of the vast majority of our gut biome health and, therefore, a profound improvement in overall quality of life can be achieved.

Prebiotics are non-digestible food ingredients that promote the growth of beneficial microorganisms in the intestines. This is a large part of the nutrition part of the jungle.

Probiotic is the actual microorganism or the plants and animals of the jungle.

Postbiotics are compounds created by bacteria that assist in the body's essential functions. This consists of the excrement and dead parts of the plants and animals.

One vital component is we can strengthen the good parts of the ecosystem by providing the right nutrients. Also, we can weaken the bad parts by not giving them their preferred foods.

The disgusting, yet unbelievable protocol is the use of fecal transplants. This is merely extracting fecal matter from thoroughly screened and healthy individuals and transferring it into the colons of unhealthy persons. The change in lives has been fascinating. This is taking an out of balance microbiome and transforming it to a healthy ecosystem.

The "avoid" food list overall contributes to the destruction of balance in the intestine. Sugar and refined flours feed candida, which has been blamed for just about every health problem in one way or another.

Dr. Ghannoum is a leader in the gut world, and his work has given me a solid foundation to decide in regard to Lander and our family's health.

Referring back to his book *The Total Gut Balance*, Dr. Ghannoum states polyphenols have antioxidant, anti-inflammatory, and anti-carcinogenic properties and have demonstrated anti-biofilm activity. Polyphenols are found in many herbs, spices, fruits, and vegetables. Two of the most well-known are curcumin and resveratrol.

Polyphenol Rich Foods:
- Green Tea
- Coffee
- Cocoa
- Onion Family (Especially Garlic)
- Turmeric
- Berries
- Nuts

Good bugs primarily eat fiber and resistant starches. This is a recurring conversation in our house. Everything we eat, we break down in a casual conversation as to how the food we are consuming affects our gut bugs. So while I'm cooking sweet potatoes, I go into how the sweet potato contains lots of good bug food.

Lander has connected that our bad bugs actually communicate with our brain. This isn't nearly as crazy as it sounds.

Although making improvements in your diet can certainly go a long way with regards to gut health, don't forget about all the other things that can affect it too.

Giving cravings for sugar and flour an identity has given us an added layer of willpower. We correlate those with bad bugs' need for them. So if our body is craving the sugar the bad bugs must be hungry and if they don't get to eat they will die. It's really worked out well for us to frame the situation in such a way that Lander has become the hero of his good bugs by feeding them and allowing them to thrive, and fighting the bad bugs by not feeding them and letting them die.

Here's a funny story about Lander and his Grandpa Joey, who Lander saw eating sugar or drinking a soft drink. He informed Grandpa Joey that by eating that way he was feeding candida. Joey looked at his wife Gina and asked, "what's candida?" Grandma Gina responded by saying Google it. They did, and pulled up images of thrush and yeast infections. It thoroughly grossed Lander's grandparents out. Just goes to show you kids really do listen to us and take to heart the things we don't always think they do.

Foods we include daily for Microbiome optimization:
- Fermented Vegetables
- Coconut Flour, Butter and Oil
- Apple Cider Vinegar
- Pecans, Pistachios and Walnuts
- Mushrooms
- Yacon Syrup

There is strong evidence extremely potent cancer fighting compounds are in soy.

(Personal note: I avoid soy for our family. I generally stay away from soy and don't allow Lander to eat it. In my estimations, the potential downside outweighs the risk. I'm always trying to learn more and may alter this decision in the future. Although any exceptions will be non-GMO and pesticide free.)

Dr. Amy Beard is a Functional Medicine practitioner as well as Board Certified Family Medicine Doctor. Before med school, she worked as a Registered Dietitian. She is someone I've come to know, respect, and trust.

I've interviewed her for our YouTube and Facebook channels about other topics, but I wanted to share what she says about the microbiome.

Dr. Amy Beard, "I keep harping on this because it's so important. Your GI tract is a HUGE part of your immune system. And its microbial inhabitants greatly influence your immune function. You have to keep those little guys happy and thriving."

Dr. Beard's list of things that negatively affect your gut health/microbiome:

1. Diets primarily consisted of processed foods, too much sugar, artificial food dyes, artificial sweeteners, low-quality seed oils, etc.
2. Medications (especially acid-suppressing meds, NSAIDs, synthetic hormones, acetaminophen, and many more)
3. Chronic stress, chronic worry
4. Inadequate sleep/lack of restorative sleep
5. Toxin exposures (current and past/cumulative effects). Too many things to list.
6. Dehydration
7. Inactivity. Yep.
8. Nutrient deficiencies
9. Tobacco products
10. Alcohol
11. Abdominal surgeries (stomach surgeries, cholecystectomies, colon resections, etc.)
12. Undiagnosed food sensitivities/intolerances

Non-Diet ways to help your gut biome:

- Get Dirty - Go outside in the fresh air and play in the dirt. Better yet play in the dirt with animals. Fresh air, sunshine and mud does the body and soul good.
- Exercise - The health benefits of exercise are extensive and help the body and mind as a whole. Bonus points if you do it outside.
- Sleep - We cover sleep much more in depth in the Practices section. Sleep helps to keep us in the cyclical means that God designed for nature. We need to make the most out of it by getting quality regular deep sleep.

Probiotic Supplements:
Dr. Gregor Reid is a Distinguished Professor of Microbiology and Immunology and Surgery at Western University, and the Endowed Chair in Human Microbiome and Probiotics at the Lawson Health Research Institute.

https://www.frontiersin.org/articles/10.3389/fmicb.2019.00424/full

Microbiome Resources:
Total Gut Balance by Dr Mahmoud Ghannoum

Podcast Transcript: Tina Anderson Co-founder Just Thrive

In this podcast, I'm joined by Tina Anderson, co-founder of Just Thrive. In addition to their flagship Probiotic, they have a full line of scientifically-backed products designed to help people feel healthy and strong.

Logan: Just Thrive is your company, and I can guarantee you it's made a significant impact on our lives, but if you don't care, introduce yourself and just a brief on how you got into this realm.

Tina: Sure, sure. Logan, thank you so much for having me. I'm glad to be here. It's such an honor to talk to you, and I love the work that you're doing by spreading the message, so keep that up. I appreciate people like you. So my story is fascinating. I started as an attorney. I was in litigation for many years. I took a very different turn. I went from litigation to have more of a desire to have more of a work-life balance. I started having children, and I wanted to have a little bit more of a work-life balance. So I went to work in our family pharmaceutical business, and I thought that was awesome because I could still practice law, but I could also help people.

I was like, this is great. We're bringing life-saving medications to people, and I was an attorney in that capacity, but I was able to have, like I said, a much better work-life balance with the kids at home. And then, after being in the industry for several years, my husband was also in the business. We just started to see a lot of abuses in the pharmaceutical industry. We saw the overprescribing of drugs. We visited relatives who would be on one medication, and the next thing you know, within a couple of months, they're on 12 different drugs and still really not getting better. And I feel strongly that there's a place for pharmaceuticals, and there's definitely a place in emergency type medicine situations or acute situations. But we didn't feel that it was a place for chronic conditions.

Instead, we thought we should focus more on getting to the root cause of an issue. My husband and I both, who started the company, read a lot of Norman Vincent Peale, Wayne Dyer. We're profound thinkers, and we didn't feel like we were doing our life's work. We didn't treat our children like this. We didn't treat our family like this. We held it off on giving an antibiotic unless it was essential. I mean, necessary. Or even if they had a fever, we didn't bring their fever down right away because we knew that that was your body's natural way of fighting an infection.

So we were looking... A lot of it was being at the right place at the right time and saying our affirmations and our prayers and meditating and all of those things. One of my husband's colleagues was able to introduce us to these incredible strains of probiotics. And we had the opportunity to license these strains of probiotics from London University, from a world-renowned probiotic expert out there. And we launched thrive probiotics. And that's how it started, and it's been the most gratifying career journey I've ever been on. No doubt.

Logan: I came across many PubMed top studies that said the effectiveness, the efficacy of a lot of chemotherapies was directed, and immunotherapies, impacted by the microbiome. So the bacteria, if we had good bacteria, could be thriving. If not, it might not. So it opened my eyes up to the microbiome. What I found with you all... I instantly bought you all are by the way. And he got it through the duration of chemo and still gets it to this day, but we don't get that bacteria now that you have in there. So can you tell us what is different about your probiotic and what was available a thousand years ago that we got naturally? And just kind of elaborate on that and why it's essential.

Tina: Yeah, and I think even if I back up, I will answer that. And then if I even back up even further to why our microbiome is so important and how it affects virtually every aspect of our overall health. And I think you hit the nail on the head. Most of the research came out not that long ago, pretty recently. The National Institutes of Health launched the Human Microbiome Project and told us more about the gut than we ever knew before. And what we found out is that the heart is responsible for virtually every single aspect of our overall health. Our immune system, like you mentioned. Our immune system, 80% of our immune system, is housed in our gut lining. So we need to have our gut microbiome, our microbiome functioning at its best so that our immune system can respond to all kinds of different pathogens that come our way, whether it be cancer, whether it be a virus, whether it be, a bacterial infection, we want our immune system a hundred percent.

And that is determined by the health of our microbiome. And the problem is that the world we live in now is so anti-microbial. We are at least 10 times more bacteria than human cells, and a challenging concept for people to understand. We are made up more of bacteria than we are of human cells. So that means... And yet, we do nothing in our world to support our bacteria that we are 10 times more of. We're not doing things. We're doing the opposite. The world we live in right now is so anti-microbial, starting with something like hand sanitizer, which I know is controversial. If I say that right now, but... Hand sanitizer is literally killing the microbes on your hands every day.

And your skin is one of your largest organs. And we need to make sure that we are... Cleaning supplies that we're using around the house, these things are killing our microbiome—antibiotics that we take, antibiotics that are found in our food. A big, colossal offender is glyphosate—the active ingredient in Roundup, which is sprayed all over our produce. So we live in this world that is attacking our microbiome daily. And then we wonder why kids have a higher incidence of cancer. Kids are having a higher incidence of autism. Kids are having a higher incidence of allergies and those types of things, auto-immune diseases. And this is why they are being raised in a much worse microbial life and world than I was even. And when I was a child, I'm much older than you are, but I knew one kid, K through 12, had a peanut allergy when I was a child.

I didn't know anybody else that had been allergic. Now, there are peanut-free tables; there's an allergy... Because it's so rampant in the world that we're living in. That's really one of the biggest things we have to understand first because we are attacking our microbiome daily, yet it's responsible for every aspect of our overall health. We said, immune system, of course. Then we talk about when you're talking about how people think of gas and bloating and diarrhea; constipation is like, "Oh, I have a gastrointestinal disturbance." You're right. That is why you would need a probiotic or why you'd need to support your gut bacteria.

But they're not thinking about, "I have anxiety or depression, or I'm feeling down, or I'm having trouble losing weight, or I'm having trouble gaining weight, or I have cancer, diabetes, or heart disease." Every one of these conditions - they are always linked to an imbalance in our gut microbiome. And that's a tricky concept for people to understand. Skin issues, people have a skin problem, and I'm like, "Oh, well, you just need to be supporting your gut microbiome." And they're like, "What does my skin have to do with my gut microbiome?" Or, "what does my mood have to do with my gut microbiome?" It has everything to do with it.

Logan: You hit on Roundup. Roundup is a pesticide, and it will be too. It acts as a pesticide also and kills bacteria. So we're not getting that bacteria from our food. It's destroyed through their pesticides and other herbicides, and we're overly clean. So you hit on that too. So all of the bacteria we, in the past, would have been ingesting is getting washed off, killed through chemicals, or just completely depleted from the environment that it's grown in, or we're killing it through cooking or processing.

Tina: Right. Exactly.

Tina: We're not getting it.

Logan: Yeah, exactly. And like you had mentioned back in the day, we used to get these bacteria, the bacteria that we're talking about, spore-based probiotics, those are the types of bacteria found in Just Thrive. But spore-based bacteria were found in the soil. These were what our ancestors used to eat daily. So they would grab their roots and tubers from the ground, and they would get those bacteria regularly. And they are not found; if you go to a tribe in Tanzania or you go to some very unpopulated area that has fresh, good, clean soil, you would get those same bacteria. And I would say, "No, you don't need to take a probiotic with spores in it." But in this situation, we don't live in that environment. Our soil, as you mentioned, it's over-farmed. It's depleted of all of the nutrients or many of the nutrients that we need. And, for sure, the probiotic that would normally naturally come from the soil.

How I describe it, it is like a bit of armadillo. So y'all's probiotics, a little armadillo, and it's balled up, and it's the shell. It doesn't have to be refrigerated. It can withstand heat. It can withstand the digestive acids in your stomach. And when it gets into the intestines where it needs to be, it opens up like a bit of armadillo and goes to work.

Tina: That's good. That's perfect.

Logan: So, is that a good analogy?

Tina: That is perfect, and that's perfect. And I think that's one of the big things that I think people are starting to understand now is that our stomach is very acidic. It's meant to be the gastric barrier. And it kills off a lot of things that go through it—a lot of the foods and something that we don't want in there. And what happens is most probiotics that are on the market actually are killed in the intestine or in the stomach acid. And they don't make it to the intestines alive. So, that's one of the biggest differences with Just Thrive is its ability to arrive alive in the intestines. And they do that exactly how you describe. It has this armor-like shell around itself when it's in its dormant state and it doesn't become alive until it hits the intestines where it takes its shell off.

And like you said, it just goes to work, working through every part of the intestinal tract. And this is a very, very different approach than the majority, overwhelming majority of probiotics that you would find in the market. Most of them are alive when they're on the shelf or in the refrigerator and that's one of the biggest myths out there about probiotics, that probiotics need to be refrigerated to stay alive. No, it needs to be refrigerated to stay alive in the refrigerator, perhaps, but it's not going to arrive alive in the intestines. And the very definition of a probiotic is "it needs to arrive alive in the intestines.". And so that's what these spores that are found at Just Thrive do very effectively. They are dormant in the bottle, in the capsule. They're not a living microorganism at the time they're dormant.

And then you swallow them. They go through your entire intestinal tract and then they go through the stomach acid, make it through the stomach acid, fine, hit the bile salts in the small intestine. And then they still are protected and it's not till they hit the intestines, they take their shell off and they go into their live vegetative cell state. And they read the microbial environment. So they're very intelligent bacteria. They're reading the bacteria. So, they're going to do something different in your intestinal tract than they will in mine, depending on where we're at. And they may produce more antibiotics to help kill off pathogenic bacteria or they may produce more nutrients to help bring certain bacteria back to life. So depending on what each of our microbiomes do. So, that's really a unique characteristic too. They're doing something very different in each of our microbiomes.

Logan: It's a powerful product, for sure. That's made a huge impact, I promise. But with the armadillo analogy, when it goes to work, that little armadillo goes to work as a gardener or whatever you want to think of it as, what is it doing? So, in terms of antioxidants, hormones, viruses, bad bacteria, what's it doing?

Tina: That's what's so cool. It does so many great things. So, in terms of pathogenic bacteria, it's going to produce a form of antibiotic to help kill off pathogenic bacteria. It's going to... When it sees good bacteria that needs to be brought back to life, it goes and helps them. It's like the garden- Actually, the best way to explain it is if you would compare it to a garden and you've got this garden that's been stepped on and trampled on. And there's weeds growing all over that garden. These go in, we're like the gardener; these strains are the gardener of the gut. They go in, they attach to the soil. So they're going to attach to the intestinal cell wall of your intestine. They're going to go, the Gardener's going to go in and get rid of the weeds in the garden.

So it's going to get rid of the pathogenic bacteria. Not all of it. It's going to kind of just rebalance it. And then it's going to go in and take those plants that have been stepped down and trampled on and help bring them back to life. And it's going to create this whole lush garden in your gut. So that's the best analogy I could use for it. The other is like if there's an overgrowth of yeast like Candida. It's kind of elbowing out the other bacteria or the overgrowth of the Candida. Candida is a natural part of our gut flora. We don't want to get rid of it entirely, but we do want to get rid of the overgrowth of it. The best way to understand these strains is not going in and blasting out things. They're not like an antimicrobial where they're going out and blasting. They're rebalancing your gut to make it a more balanced and healthier environment. We are doing great things for all of those things.

Logan: Well, thank you. Thank you for what you're doing in the work and the education. We appreciate the education and your willingness to get out and teach people. At its base, I think that's probably the most important thing that we're able to do daily for overall health.

Tina: Well, yeah. Like you had said... First of all, thank you for doing the health. I have been so blessed to know so many health food store owners and managers and aisle clerks who are just so knowledgeable. Sometimes they're more knowledgeable than my doctors, you know? And I go to pretty cool doctors but functional medicine and all of that. But I think that health food store owners, you are really, they take it so seriously. And I love that. And I think that's why people trust you guys so much because you do the research and take the time to do things like you're doing right now, listening to other podcasts and growing your knowledge base. So kudos to you. But I do... When you mentioned that about cancer treatments and chemo being better absorbed by having a healthy microbiome that goes with anything. People could eat this clean diet and kale and broccoli and organic foods and spinach and all these great and really healthy nutrient-dense foods.

But if your gut is inflamed in any way and your gut is not, it's not absorbing those nutrients; you could be taking supplements like crazy. But if your gut is inflamed and your microbiome is not the healthiest it could be, it's not absorbing those nutrients as effectively. So I always feel that this is ground zero. It used to be, years ago, people would say, "Oh, I'm going to at least take a multivitamin." And while there is undoubtedly an argument for a multivitamin, we need to make sure that whatever we're taking is being absorbed by our microbiome. And so that's why we must start number one; if there's one supplement someone's going to take, it would be a spore-based probiotic. That is the number one ground zero for health.

The other thing you mentioned, I forgot to answer, is you said about antioxidants; one of the strains in our product produces RDA levels of antioxidants in the gut. So it's producing alpha beta carotene, lycopene, lutein, astaxanthin, zeaxanthin; all these incredible antioxidants are being made right in the gut exactly where they need to be absorbed. So one of the most bioavailable forms of antioxidants, which is great for the gut lining and supporting the health of our gut lining. I appreciate the opportunity. I admire people like you that have those big audacious goals to make a difference in the world, and you're going to do it. You're already doing it. Such a great job. Thank you. And lots of prayers to your son, to your whole family, and good for you for making good out of it.

Just Thrive products are an absolute cornerstone of the Landerman Plan and can be found in Lander's Corner and can be purchased at JustThriveHealth.com

Use code LanderMan for a discount!

Farmer's Market Connection

The common denominator in health is diet. This is where farmer's markets can make a massive impact by providing access and education of a wide range of fruits, vegetables and meat.

Locally sourced produce should have a higher nutrient profile. This gives those who consume it a step ahead of mass-produced foods. Especially in the much shorter distance, the fresh produce travels.

Food is medicine and it's not fully understood all of the benefits of a whole foods diet, but for those who adhere to one, they tend to be significantly healthier.

From a nutrient overview, a Paleo Diet is high in fiber, medium in fats, lower in animal proteins, and low in sugar-based carbohydrates. Due to the consumption of a large amount of plant material, our ancestors consumed high in fiber, smaller portions of meat and eggs, and consequently a lower percentage of animal-based protein. Think of meat as more of a condiment than a star of the meal, and small amounts of seasonal fruits. Depending on the geographic location, fats from plants also made up a significant part of the diet from a wide variety of nuts, coconuts, avocados, olives, and cocoa.

I love that the Paleo Diet is simple and focuses on the quality of the foods. Processed foods are entirely against the fundamental principle of Paleo. The modern equivalent of a Paleo Diet is grass-fed and pastured meats from beef, bison, sheep, pork, goat and poultry. Plant-based organic and naturally grown foods lead to avoiding modern cultivated crops with GMO and pesticide components.

What is a Ketogenic Diet or Keto?

Overall a Ketogenic Diet is straightforward in its broad definition; it is very low in carbohydrates. Probably the most famous Keto Diet is the Atkins Diet.

The low amount of carbs leads to the conversion of fats by the liver into ketones instead of utilizing glucose for fuel in cellular function. This process and the science behind it can get complicated pretty quickly.

Keto has helped a lot of people drop excess weight and has changed lives, but the long-term effects are significant.

Dirty Keto is a version focused strictly on the macro view of limiting carbs. Therefore, as long as it's low or no-carb, it's good to go. Without getting too far into it, I think we can all agree this isn't healthy, especially long term, hence the name "Dirty Keto."

A significant division within keto is whether to get calories from fats or proteins. For the standard American diet, it is a much smoother transition to a high protein side.

In developing an eating plan for Lander to optimize his health and attempt to negate the ill effects of chemo and other accompanying treatments, I've looked extensively into the ketogenic diet among many, many others. There are numerous beneficial components.

When you combine principles of Paleo and Keto, you get a powerful coupling and what I refer to as Clean Keto. Many of the principles inside that philosophy make up the core of how we eat.

There is an additional layer of emphasis on a few physiologically specific components. The microbiome is an integral part of the plan, and everything is viewed through a systematic approach considering gut health.

Health Team:

Fitness is also an extremely important part of health and life. Regular exercise absolutely is one of the top contributors to optimal health.

Stress Management is a practice for which many of us are guilty of neglecting by saying we don't have the time. High stress levels come from a lack of spending time doing things like exercising, taking walks in a park, meditating, and doing yoga, to name a few. These are activities that aid in dealing with the fast-paced, crazy life many of us live.

Functional Medicine:

The further I've gotten into this journey, the more I appreciate Functional Medicine. Oftentimes, the western model of medicine focuses mainly on the symptoms.

For example, when we have a headache we normally go to our medicine cabinet and take a pill, (aspirin or analgesic, for example). That's focusing on the symptoms. Functional Medicine, by contrast, wants to discover and uncover why we have the headache in the first place. Is it a sinus infection, or an impacted tooth? Do we have any muscles causing a nerve to be pinched? It's just a more in-depth way of looking at resolving the core issue.

One of the largest impacts I've seen are in the way Functional Medicine deals with gut issues and pain. At our farmer's market, I hear people having issues, for example, with constipation. Most medical experts will tell them to take a laxative or eat more fiber. In contrast, a Functional Medicine practitioner would likely run lab tests and look at lab values differently than that of their western counterparts. For example, many times looking at thyroid levels to include reverse T3 that many times is overlooked, or perhaps another microbiome condition, or even some sort of a food sensitivity like that of gluten.

The point of all this is to indicate that Functional Medicine practitioners tend to look at the whole body and not be over specialized. Western medicine practitioners often refer their patients to an endocrinologist, a gastroenterologist, a neurologist, optometrist, dermatologist, and many other specialists that don't necessarily work together in any facet.

Integrative Oncology - If you or someone you know has cancer, I recommend the podcast *Cancer Secrets - Integrative Oncologist*, Jonathan Stegall, MD.

Cancer is by many evaluations, "the perfect disease". I know that may sound crazy, but it is a disease that has so many fronts, all of which we must face. Cancer will beat us if we are unable to holistically correct the wide range of facets from nutrients, immune system, mindset, gut microbiome and so many more.

Farmer's markets offer the opportunity to bring together a hub of people who, in my experience, care about health, quality food, the environment, and the community. By connecting specialists and groups, farmer's markets have a significant impact on community health.

Additionally, visiting a farmer's market should be that of a positive experience. This naturally should help reduce stress.

Podcast Transcript: Wade Lightheart, CEO/Founder of BiOptimizer

I visited with Wade Lightheart, CEO and Founder of *BiOptimizer*. He discussed health issues and pointed out a major connection to farming.

Logan: Can you tell us why we may be seeing this epidemic of gut problems?

Wade Lightheart: Great question. It's the unintended consequences of technological innovation. And so you have to go back in time. If you go back before world war, when World War II happened, the United States dropped the nuclear bomb on Japan, finally ending the war. The Japanese surrendered that war shortly afterward and the baby boom happened. And all of a sudden there was an explosion of the population all around the world. And the governments of the world started to recognize that the old patterns of farming and people moving to the city and stuff, wouldn't be able to supply a sufficient amount of food to the population. So they got well-meaning boards and regulatory boards and agricultural boards and these things of what we needed to do.

And what was implemented in short order in the next little while was monoculturing farming.

And when monocultural farming came in, prior to that, farming for thousands of years involved, a thing called crop rotation. You grow your crops, you grow tomatoes here one year and you grow squash here the following year, and you grow potatoes the next year and then you have one year where you grow hemp and then you plow that hemp back into the ground to reconstitute the soil and you let the soil go fallow. And if you go out to the West, out into Western Canada, for example, I'm from Canada. You'll actually see the big farms. They'll have one little section, which is where the farmers used to eat their food. And then they had the mono culturing one. Many that were subsidized and government-sponsored programs. And then what began to happen as the soil's mineral content went down, they couldn't grow the crops fast enough, they would yield. So they used the leftover nitrogen from all the bombs that were irrelevant and leftover from the war to put the nitrogen on the soil. Now what happens? We put the nitrogen on the soil, it grows the vegetables and fruits much faster.

However, you give up essential amino acids, you give up enzymes and you have less vitamins and minerals within that food. These proteins are very important for the health and durability of the plant, whether it's how hardy that plant is and how resistant it is to disease and bugs and things like that. So after a few generations of that, all of a sudden, various types of diseases started to wipe out entire crops. Blights and of course, insurance agencies started to get crop protection and all these sorts of things. So there were industries built out of this. But long story short, the chemical company said, "Well, hey, well, let's add herbicides, pesticides, and fungicides to the food onto the vegetables and stuff. So that came into Vogue and the various chemical plants and fertilizers in the marketing campaigns that came on it now. So, how those chemicals work is they interrupt the natural enzymatic activity of the bugs of the organism they're trying to kill.

So much so, that it will kill them. And enzymes are the difference between the living and the dead between stones, plants, and people. And you have, what's called an enzyme bank account. And this is well illustrated by a fellow by the name of Dr. Edward Howell, who wrote enzyme nutrition and food enzymes for health and longevity. And he determined back then by doing all these different species for checking out all these different species, dogs, cats, rats, you name it. And he found that if you fed them an enzymatically deficient diet over three generations number one, they started to exert a massive amount of genetic based diseases, number two, they started to elicit strange sociological behaviors, and number three, the species lost the ability to procreate. Well, fast forward, it's been three generations since we implemented these components in the world. And we see all of those three playing out in the human population just yeah, as Howell suggested.

So my mentor was a guy by the name of Dr. Michael O'Brien and he was instrumental in helping Bernard Jensen overcome cancer at the end of his life. And Bernard even wrote the book on digestive health. A lot of people don't know that in his book, his last book I think was called *Come Alive*, which documents he dedicated it to Dr. O'Brien, and he explained to him a little bit about some of the things that he used to implement in order to keep his recovery. I want to be clear about something. I'm not suggesting that enzymes and probiotics can help a person or what will cause the recovery from a serious illness. What I'm saying is, is the deficiency in these elemental components, which are a natural part of our food supply throughout all history are now devoid, thanks to chemicalization, irradiation, judging and processing, that occurs with our food supply chain, not to mention all the foods that are manufactured completely artificially.

So when you do this, disrupt your digestive system. Now, let's look at the statistics that are out there. 12% of the emergency hospital visits in this country are related to gastrointestinal-related illnesses, a hundred million people on any given day have some sort of digestive discomfort. And over 25% of those people are on prescription medication. So medication is always just a way to mitigate the symptoms of a disease because oftentimes, the causes are unknown or are multi-varied in their factors. And what I would say to any person who is experiencing any sort of digestive distress, weight gain, over an excessive healthy body weight, they have to address the lifestyle issues that are related to, or even the extreme case, some sort of metabolic or disease-based condition. And what I would suggest to people. And this is the theory that we put forward, and that is health and disease are the natural result of the environmental conditions, both internally and externally of that given individual over the genetic predispositions present in that organism.

So some people have a predisposition for heart disease. Some people have a predisposition to cancer. Some people who have a predisposition for whatever, but what we are seeing is a dramatic, insignificant rise in gastro-related illnesses. Now that's where your food goes into the body. Your food goes, it goes into the body. You know, there's a process of digestion, absorption, and assimilation. Basically, it's a five-stage process that involves, from tasting, touching, chewing the food, going into the esophagus, down into the stomach, hydrochloric acid, coming in, disinfecting it, minerals coming in, buffering the acids. Then that travels down to the gut where the good guys and the bad guys left, and hopefully have more good guys than bad guys. And then they convert what's leftover that food into the energy units or the building blocks of your body.

A failure on any part in one area of that, the insufficient enzymes insufficient hydrochloric acid, an unbalance in the microbiome will result in digestive distress, left unchecked over time, this will compromise that person's health, their vitality, their energy, and increase the likelihood that they will suffer from the devastating effects of either a life like a permanent disability in disease or the loss of life itself. And so, our whole mission is to kind of bring people well to the awareness that getting your digestion working properly so that you can assimilate the good things that you're going to eat and get rid of the bad things as an essential component in conjunction with a healthy lifestyle and a healthy diet.

Enzyme is a worker in your body, same as the workers in your local town that clean the streets and keep the power on, and the plumbing working and the streets plowed in the snow and fix the power wires. They are the workers of the body. They are chemical catalysts. Basically, virtually every chemical reaction in the body requires an enzyme. And what it does is it turns one thing into something else. And these chemical processes are all through the body. There's over 25,000 inside the human body that they know of. And they seem like they keep discovering more and more. Now when it comes to, there's different enzymatic pathways, proteolytic pathways, which are related to proteins, glycolytic pathways, which are related to carbohydrates, and lipolytic pathways, which are related to fats. Basically there are enzymes that are involved in various chains, not only just from digestion, but also inside the body.

And so these catalysts are kind of like, it's like a bank account. When you're born, you have so much money, you have inherited a chemical or an enzymatic bank account. And that's how Dr. Hal put it. And any woman who has had several children will tell you, they do not have the same life force and energy they had before the kids. They actually deposit a great chunk of their enzymatic activity to the child. And so this determines how many metabolic checks, chemical checks you can write in your life. Now, every species on the planet keeps getting enzymes because they eat their food in a live, raw state. Whether it's a tiger eating animals, whether it's a horse or a cow eating grass, whether it's a bear, eating salmon and blueberries, they all get it. And all living things have enzymes. So not only do you get the proteins, carbohydrates, fats, or whatever nutrients are here, but you get the enzymes, but that wasn't defined in our food.

Now we cook our food. We irradiate our food. We spray our food and we deplete the enzymatic count. So what happens is our body has to manufacture these enzymes itself at huge metabolic costs. That's why you get so tired after having the giant Thanksgiving dinner with the turkey and the potatoes and all this stuff, I call the Turkey. Everybody goes, passes out because your body says, "I don't have enough of these workers to run my brain right now. I don't have enough to run my muscles right now. I'm going to take all of my enzyme production just to break down the food." And then once we've got that, you know, Uncle Joe wakes up from drooling on the couch and Grandma snaps out of it from snoring in the chair. And you know, little Linda, she gets up off the floor after passing out and drooling all over her face and they go for another round.

So there is a conversion process of turning your food into the energy and building block, which requires enzymes. I say everything from thinking to blinking requires enzymes. So when a person's enzymatic bank account is lower than it can write checks and the demands from life, whether that's from performance, sports, like I was involved, whether it's from disease, whether it's from stress, whatever it happens to be that causes you to, you need to write more checks, what happens is if you don't have enough, your body will start shutting down different operational components. We call that aging in degeneration, but it's been accelerated in the population so that now kids are getting diseases that were originally designed for senior citizens.

So eating the American diet, you're not getting any enzymes.

There's a fellow by the name of Dr. Gonzalez who took super physiological doses of enzymes. And this is well-documented over 12,000 cases and people with extreme levels of, of disease and cancer in particular. And he was able to elicit the recovery in many of those people. Now people go, is it the enzymes that did that? No, I wouldn't say that. I would say what the enzymes allowed a body to do is write more metabolic checks. And by doing that, if you're doing everything else, right, and you're following all the things that you need to do, and God willing, then you are able to do things that your medical advisors might not be aware of.

Not saying that they're wrong. I'm not saying they're doing the best that they can with what they have been given, but they are not experts in this field. And I'm certainly not suggesting that you can go out and cure all these different diseases from whatever. I'm not saying that what

I'm saying is, is the bottom line is when you get sick or you've been sick or you want to prevent being sick, it all comes down to your lifestyle and how you're going to address it and recognize that because of the technological innovations of the world, fact that we can talk on the internet and flying planes and driving cars, well, we're very unique in the human story, in the human history. And there are consequences to these conveniences that we didn't anticipate when we created them.

Logan: Absolutely, absolutely. So with, with that, it's our bodies giving it what it needs, taking away the things it doesn't, so toxicities and whatever that means, given what our bodies can do some pretty amazing things on their own.

Wade Lightfoot: Healing and disease I believe are, or health and disease are the natural results of internal and external conditions, overtop of the biochemistry of that particular organism. And it's really important to understand that. And so, one of the tendencies, and one of the things I want to comment on is when you talked about this at first. As devastating as that situation to have your child sick, and I've witnessed my parents go through it and many, many others, you can take on the role of a victim of it, or you can take on the role of a victor. That does not guarantee the outcome. It only guarantees that you are going to take up the fight with everything that you have. And I think it's important for people to really do their due diligence and go above and beyond to support whatever your medical professionals are suggesting and recommending.

Logan: Absolutely. I agree with that wholeheartedly. I used to get really frustrated when western medical doctors, who I have a lot of friends, and are wonderful people, were either dismissive of a lot of the natural ways or nutrition, but then the more I've looked into it that they legitimately don't know. Whether that's on purpose or not, it's not for me to say, but that's why, what we are doing I feel is so unbelievably important. So Arkansas is typically like 48th, 49th on unhealthiest States in the United States, like consistently in horrible, horrible health. So, that awareness is what we want to do. We have, I have doctors come to me and we have conversations on how to incorporate these types of things. You know, it's just that awareness and brother you coming on here and just sharing with our audience, means so much because you an absolute expert when it comes to the digestion and supplements space.

People are fed by the food industry, which pays no attention to health, and are treated by the health industry, which pays no attention to food. ♥ Wendell Berry

---

Recommended Supplements:

As with any health advice, it's best to work with a professional to help guide you. Bloodwork and one on one conversations are essential to stay on top of maintaining good health. Everyone is different, therefore I highly recommend having a functional medicine physician to guide you on your journey to discovering optimum health.

The gut-wrenching moment I heard the word *cancer* spoken in reference to the health and well-being of my very own child, I vowed then and there to embark on a boundless battle plan, and search high and low for every single resource available to mankind to save my son from the clutches of that horrific disease.

To say that I have learned so much along the way would be a profound understatement. Doors have been opened, searches have been successful, and astounding, caring and knowledgeable people have entered my life.

Here is an excellent article https://www.healthline.com/nutrition/optimize-omega-6-omega-3-ratio#section1

The LanderMan Plan significantly helps to balance the ratio. Another way we help to ensure it is by eating grass fed meat, eggs and butter, taking supplements and avoiding oils like vegetable and canola oils which are in a vast array of products.

My two older children, Lander and Kamry, get algae spray that is lemon-flavored and the babies get drops. Nordic Naturals has been a great brand in my experience.

My current favorite addition to my supplement list includes taking krill oil capsules. The krill oil is less likely to be contaminated by heavy metals such as mercury. It also contains Astaxanthin, an orange-pinkish carotenoid extensively found in marine organisms and has numerous health-benefiting properties.

If you want to get deep into the science, here is a great article https://www.ncbi.nlm.nih.gov/pmc/articles/PMC3967194/

There are plenty of deficiencies we can cover in depth but I personally haven't see the first-hand improvement by a large amount of people like I have with magnesium.

Magnesium is massively depleted in our diet. The mineral is vital for over 300 functions within the body.

BiOptimizers has a full line up of incredible products and has a formula of "7 Forms of Magnesium Transforms Your Stress & Performance."

One of the biggest misconceptions about magnesium is that you just "need more" of it and you'll be healthy and optimized.

But there are many different magnesium types — and each plays a critical role in different functions in your body.

Most "healthy" people only get 1-2 forms at best (much of the population is deficient in all forms) — but when you get all 7 major forms of magnesium, that's when the magic happens.

MAGNESIUM CHELATE - This form of magnesium is especially important for muscle building, recovery, and health.

MAGNESIUM CITRATE - Helps with the effects of obesity. One study found that this form helped arterial stiffness in healthy overweight individuals.

MAGNESIUM BISGLYCINATE - Often used to treat excess stomach acid symptoms, such as stomach upset, heartburn, and acid indigestion.

MAGNESIUM MALATE - Some believe this to be the most bioavailable form of magnesium. It's found naturally in fruits, giving them a "tart taste." Magnesium Malate can help with migraines, chronic pain, and depression.

MAGNESIUM SUCROSOMIAL - This form of magnesium helps you to produce energy effectively. It also supports the immune system and is critical for bone health and skeletal development.

MAGNESIUM TAURATE - This is the form of magnesium best for your heart.

MAGNESIUM OROTATE -While also helpful for the heart, magnesium orotate is believed to be the best form for metabolic improvements.

Magnesium Breakthrough has been found in Lander's Corner as one of the first supplements and has remained a constant repurchase because of the impact it is making.

BiOptimizers, as Wade Lightherat explained in our visit, has an enzyme product that aids in digestion but has secondary benefits in overall health. I can't recommend enzymes enough.

Turmeric kept coming up repeatedly in my research as a critical component in alleviating a considerable range of negative effects, and most importantly to my family are the anticancer properties.

Curcumin has been referenced in a ton of published research studies, and so many of the claims can be scientifically substantiated.

Ultra Botanica has developed a product, *UltraCur,* that gets the highest known amount of curcuminoids into the blood, maximizing effects.

They have also developed a superfoods green drink mix, UltraBoost containing the UltraCur product and the main drink I use for Lander.

Probiotics are the good bugs that live in our intestines. The microbiome is one of the rabbit trails I went down that crossed every health area and became more and more evidence of its importance.

The gut microbiome is easily destroyed by antibiotics, pesticides, medications, and poor nutrition. It's a lot like any other ecosystem in that there needs to be a balance. Viruses, bacteria, and fungi all live within the body and have roles to play. Problems arise when a good player isn't present, or a bad guy grows out of hand.

Research shows the vast majority of our body's immune function is located, or originates, in the gut. Additionally, with regards to cancer, the effectiveness of some chemotherapy and immunotherapies is partially dependent on the microbiome being optimized.

There are massive amounts of probiotic supplements on the market. In the grand scheme of things, the area is still in its infancy, and we don't know what all we don't know.

Just Thrive is my favorite product line. I gave Lander their "Probiotic and Antioxidant" formula during his chemo and radiation treatments and he continues to take it on a regular basis. In fact, I have my entire family on this regimen.

The probiotic spore-based bacteria are like the ones found in the soil. Our ancestors ate these on a regular basis, especially from root crops like carrots, beets, and potatoes that weren't overly clean.

That's right, too clean isn't healthy. Are you surprised to learn that? I was too.

Lander's page on the Just Thrive website is at https://justthrivehealth. com/landerman and use code LanderMan for a discount!

Beam Minerals, humic and fulvic acid, is a product I've fallen in love with. My only regret is I didn't discover it earlier in our journey. Again, thanks to the work of Dave Asprey and Bulletproof Radio, I became aware of this life changing product.

As a source of essential minerals, amino acids, electrolytes, and antioxidants, humic and fulvic acid are an easy way for the body to get needed components to address potential deficiencies.

On the toxicity topic, Beam Minerals are a natural chelator of toxins like heavy metals and have detoxification effects. All in all, improving cellular function and overall health.

As with all of the supplements I fully believe in, I contact and work directly with them. No one knows their own product and mission like the source.

Caroline Alan, Co-Founder of Beam Minerals offered a discount code Lander on their website.

These core supplements cover a broad base and aren't overly specialized to which have negative effects. Always work with a healthcare professional and follow their guidance or the instruction accompanying the product.

Health and Nature:

Spending time in nature is a beautiful way to embrace health in an inexpensive way.

Many people don't breathe fresh air, aren't exposed to natural light, and don't get fresh dirt on them. All of which lead to major health benefits.

The first way nature helps is with light. We are unbelievably dependent on light with different wavelengths.

Digging and playing in the dirt are extremely beneficial - especially out in the sunshine.

Don't be afraid to take off your shoes and walk on the grass or better yet the beach. Grounding is the practice that is gaining a lot of traction and for good reason.

Stress Management - Nutrients, Foods, and Acupuncture

Life can be stressful, but we can manage it in lots of ways. As I write this, we have just overcome an unprecedented Arkansas snowstorm after a heated presidential election cycle during the COVID pandemic. Outside stress from relationships, finances, and employment can become compounded in addition to internal stress of illness for many.

How does stress affect the body?

Not all stress is harmful and is a natural part of human survival. In a sudden dangerous situation, the increased heart rate, rapid breath, and tensed muscles push more oxygen to the brain increasing our ability to fight off the stressor. Having these quick responses improves our outcomes in life-or-death situations.

However, over the long term, major health problems arise and can affect everything from sleep, appetite, irritability, and even headaches, with constant stress. With extended periods of stress, the immune system becomes depressed and causes spikes in blood sugar levels. Prolonged or chronic stress is associated with severe conditions like diabetes, depression, and heart disease. Also, vital nutrients are used rapidly and become extremely low.

What nutrients are depleted, and where do we get them?

Micronutrients are vital for optimal health. We know vitamins C and D play crucial roles in the immune system. Minerals such as zinc, magnesium, and calcium also have significant impacts on our health.

Research out of Australia shows these five essential nutrients are depleted.

1. Magnesium
2. Vitamin C
3. Vitamin B5
4. Vitamin B6
5. Zinc

Magnesium and zinc are common deficiencies, to begin with, and with stress, it is even more crucial to make sure adequate amounts are included in diet or by supplementation.

What are some stress-fighting foods?

Herbal teas such as lavender and chamomile are known for reducing anxiety and helping people fall asleep. They are also used to calm an upset stomach and other digestive issues.

Dark Chocolate is actually healthy food. Cocoa is an antioxidant and polyphenol powerhouse. Sugar and milk are what take away from such an extraordinary indulgence. Cortisol is the body's main stress hormone which is very important in a wide range of functions with blood sugar, blood pressure, sleep cycle, and more. Excessively high levels for extended periods of time can cause major problems. There is evidence regular consumption of dark chocolate results in less cortisol being released into the body.

Avocados are another great addition to the arsenal of stress-fighting foods. They are loaded with good fats like omega 3's, phytochemicals, fiber, and other essential nutrients.

Gut health and microbiome are always the core of our focus. Supplementing with probiotics and prebiotics are ways to boost mood with serotonin and gamma-aminobutyric acid (GABA). The hormone serotonin stabilizes our mood and impacts happiness as well as affects the entire body, enabling brain cells and other nervous system cells to communicate with each other.

Other ways to manage stress:

Adaptogens are plant and mushroom products that counteract the effects of stress in the body.

Supplements https://www.healthline.com/health/stress/smart-girls-guide-to-adaptogens#how-to-use-adaptogens

- Ashwagandha
- Rhodiola
- Cordyceps
- Turmeric

Exercise and movement are tremendous stress reducers. They offer a multitude of health benefits. When Lander was in the middle of the treatments and the unknowns began to suffocate my thoughts, going to the gym was a significant way for me to work through the stress. I honestly believe it was one of the most significant contributors to keeping me level-headed.

Sunshine is quite possibly the most overlooked contributor to health. This is a topic I will go into in much more depth in the future—the different wavelengths of light act in many ways with the body. The most common way is the production of Vitamin D. Still, many more types are being studied such as early morning light and the effects on melatonin production in the evening and night.

Sleep is another topic deserving of its own article. A great book I recommend is *The Power of When* by Dr. Micheal Breus. Sleep helps us reset and recover.

Healing Points Acupuncture Clinic - North Little Rock, Arkansas

Michele Fincher was born and raised in Little Rock, Arkansas, and has been a licensed acupuncturist and herbalist since 2009. She earned a Bachelor of Arts in Social Work from the University of Arkansas and a Master of Science in Traditional Chinese Medicine Degree from the American College of Traditional Chinese Medicine in San Francisco, California. In addition, Michele has also received advanced clinical training in Hangzhou, China from the Zhejiang Medical University.

Michele's private practice clinic, Healing Points Acupuncture, is in Downtown North Little Rock in the Argenta Arts District. She treats a variety of health conditions and offers individualized care to patients of all ages.

Acupuncture is probably a scary or uncomfortable thought for most. I hope to demystify the ancient practice. I took my film crew to the acupuncture clinic run by my friend, Michele Fincher, L.Ac., Dipl. OM to document her providing one of her patients with an acupuncture treatment. While we were there, I visited with her about the positive health benefits of acupuncture:

How can acupuncture help caregivers and cancer patients deal with stress?

The benefits of acupuncture for cancer patients reach far and wide. But it can also do wonders for those who are taking care of cancer patients. Many find acupuncture to be a crucial part of their self-care regimen.

Acupuncture restores the body's stress equilibrium by inserting very thin needles along energy pathways in the body to stimulate the body's innate healing ability. For thousands of years acupuncture has been used to help prevent disease, treat illness, and improve overall well-being. It treats the mind, body and spirit and views each structure in your body as an integral and necessary part of the whole.

Acupuncture can be a great stress reducer for any cancer patient. Cancer patients who use acupuncture report they feel calmer and happier. They also claim to feel more mentally alert and emotionally stable.

Learning that a loved one has been diagnosed with cancer can be one of the most stressful things for someone to experience. As a caregiver, you must be a rock for the person suffering with the disease and you must be there to support them physically, mentally, and emotionally. That is a heavy burden for someone who is dealing with the fact that someone they love is undergoing what is most likely going to be the hardest part of their life.

Acupuncture can proactively reduce stress in the following ways:

1. By creating balance in the Nervous System. Acupuncture works by stimulating the Central Nervous System. This releases natural endorphins into the body like serotonin that help calm responses to stress by lowering cortisol levels which will increase under stress.

2. By providing much needed respite for caregivers and cancer patients alike and it creates scheduled time for rest and self-care. Acupuncture is relaxing and makes you feel good! It is not scary nor painful.

3. By boosting your own energy naturally which stress can deplete.

4. By reducing inflammation which can lead to many different types of illness, both mental and physical. Acupuncture is inherently stress reducing and has a distinctly overall calming effect which lowers inflammation. The more consistently the treatment is given the greater the cumulative effect.

5. By providing ongoing physical, mental, and emotional support. Acupuncturists also remind you of other ways to reduce stress too, such as breathing, movement, hydration, nutrition, sleep, laughter, and gratitude. Remember to count your blessings!

Acupuncture is a safe and effective treatment

When performed by a trained and licensed professional acupuncture is extremely safe. It is a natural, non-drug therapy and is virtually side effect free and has helped people for centuries to reduce stress and improve health and wellness. Every patient is unique and so are their health concerns. At Healing Points Acupuncture we take this into consideration and treat patients accordingly by identifying imbalances in the body through pulse and tongue diagnosis.

In most cases it is not the stress that is the problem, but how you react to the stress.

Acupuncture is an effective therapy for the treatment of stress and anxiety disorders. Acupuncture redirects your qi (pronounced chee) or vital life force energy into a more balanced flow helping to resolve the cause and effects of stress in your body. Acupuncture releases tension in the muscles and this allows increased flow of blood, lymph, and nerve impulses to affected areas, thus decreasing the stress experienced by the patient.

If you or anyone you know is experiencing emotional or physical distress from an illness or from caregiving acupuncture is a very effective treatment.

Biohacking

*"The art and science of changing the environment
around you and inside you so that you have full
control over your own biology."* Dave Asprey

Sleep

To say it was hard to sleep when Lander was diagnosed with cancer
would be a massive understatement. I don't know that I slept for the first
week or two after that. The importance of sleep is pretty evident from
my years of working on an ambulance and going without it and the toll
it would take trying to push through days.

I knew I needed to be the best for Lander and my family so it was
evident I would need to figure out how to get sleep even though it was
extremely difficult. I began tracking my sleep, and experimenting, while
researching how to improve sleep, and the non-stop searching for ways
to help my child. It was a merry-go-round.

All biological systems are cyclical. To best perform, we must allow our bodies the opportunity to recover. The cyclical way our bodies recover is through quality sleep. This section can't be stressed enough.

Sleep is infinitely complex, and in many ways, the field of study hasn't scratched the surface. Two excellent resources to go in-depth are *"Why We Sleep"* by Matthew Walker, Ph.D. and *"The Power of When"* by Dr. Michael Breus.

It is essential to note higher quality sleep is more important than more sleep. The 3 phases of sleep are light - which is useless, Deep, and REM.

Deep sleep is the rejuvenating phase of sleep in which muscles grow and repair. A relatively recent discovery is that of the glymphatic system, which uses cerebral spinal fluid to wash the brain, flushing wastes, and neurotoxins. This system activates in the Deep Sleep phase. It is highly likely a link between the uptick in dementia and Alzheimers is in part related to poor quality sleep and nutrition.

REM (Rapid Eye Movement) is the re-energizing phase of sleep associated with dreaming, memory retention, learning, and creativity.

The only way to fully understand our sleep is to monitor it. Many bracelets and other devices have methods of analyzing sleep. I use the Oura ring, and much prefer it over a band.

Sleep Tips
Oral Hygiene - this may seem obvious, but brushing your teeth before bed has a significant effect on sleep quality.

1. Don't eat before bed - a great rule of thumb is don't eat after dark. While this may sound extreme, it's not.
2. Consistent bedtime. Try to have a relatively narrow window (Within 90 minutes) in which you go to sleep.

3. Stay away from blue light at least an hour before bed. Blue lights disrupt melatonin production leading to poor quality sleep and trouble falling asleep. Install a blue light blocker app on the phone.
4. Proper nutrition and supplementation play a massive part.
   a. Vitamin D
   b. Magnesium
   c. Collagen
   d. Herbal Teas
5. Dark room or sleep mask
6. Weighted Blanket

Skincare

Cancer is the reason I've dove into most of the research aspects of health. Skin is no exception. Remembering back to my grandfather and all of the cancer patients I encountered working on in ambulances, they all had some sort of issue with sensitive, dry cracked and even peeling skin.

Skin is extremely important for overall health. It helps regulate body temperature and is the barrier making it the first-line protection in the immune system.

Early on when Lander began treatments, I wanted to stay ahead of problems. I first looked at what caused the negative conditions.

What causes dry skin for cancer patients?

Dry skin is caused by many things especially for cancer patients, and treatment is often the major contributor.

Chemotherapy and radiation can disrupt this process of rapidly dividing cells. This is great when targeting cancer, but also damages and destroys other cells like hair, skin, and other epithelial tissue like the inside of the mouth and nose. This process causes dry skin and other skin issues, even sores.

The goal of radiation is to target cancer cells. It causes the skin to be dry, flaky, and in some cases leads to burns.

What I Did for Lander?

The first thing I did with Lander was to get oils to apply to his body. I got a combination of Jojoba and Vitamin E oil. Then, I added Almond oil later in the process. Every time Lander took a bath, I would add the oil mix and Epsom salt.

After the bath, we put the oil all over his body, even his head when he lost all of his hair. I took special care to keep oil directly on his incisions and port. His scars, considering the extent and size, healed very well.

Often nurses commented on how good Lander's port site looked. A port is a needle access point surgically placed under the skin. They are necessary due to the continued need to start IV, draw blood, and save excessive needle sticks which leads to destroyed veins.

That nightly routine obviously made a positive impact. The other aspect of skincare was the use of red and near-infrared light therapy. The machine I got was the Joovv. https://joovv.com/blogs/joovv-blog/why-use-red-light-therapy

Natural sunlight is very important and the full spectrum light adds benefits to overall health. Lander was encouraged to play outside not only for sunlight exposure, but also for exercise.

Different wavelengths do an array of things like promoting healthy mitochondria function, which produces cellular energy, and also helps build collagen, and studies show it reduces inflammation.

After the positive results with the oil, I teamed up with Keri Miller of Beauty from Ashes to create a standard blend. After continued research and experimentation we settle on a Jojoba base with Vitamin E, Almond, and Rosehip Oils. We named the blend Rednal Oil which is Lander spelled backwards.

Nightly Routine with Lander

- Bath with Epsom Salt, Jojoba and Vitamin E oil
- Oil directly over his port and scars
- Joovv Red Light Machine

Lander's tumor was the size of a cantaloupe and his entire kidney was removed. Chemo, contrast used for scans and dehydration can be hard on kidneys. For those reasons making sure he drank plenty of fluids daily was a focus. The added benefit helped keep his skin healthy.

Foods for skin

1. Fish – Salmon and Mackerel are my favorites. They are loaded with Omega 3's, vitamins and minerals.
2. Green Tea – polyphenols and carotenoids contribute to improved skin function. https://pubmed.ncbi.nlm.nih.gov/21525260/
3. Dark Chocolate – Phytochemicals protect the skin form UV radiation https://pubmed.ncbi.nlm.nih.gov/25116848/
4. Sweet Potatoes – High in beta carotene which is the precursor to Vitamin A
5. Avocados – Loaded with good fats, vitamins E and C.

Action Steps

1. Abide by a clean diet plan - Everyone is different but these are great starts. All of them have very similar fundamentals.
   a. *Bulletproof* - Dave Asprey - More Ketogenic, Gluten Free
   b. *Pegan* - Dr Mark Hyman - Between Vegan and Paleo
   c. *Wahls Protocol* - Dr Terry Wahls - Highly Recommend for Autoimmune
   d. *Longevity Diet* - Dr Valter Longo - Also includes fasting
   e. *Blue Zone Kitchen* - Dan Buettner - Includes Fruits, Beans and Starchy Vegetables
2. Move everyday, get outside, and walk in nature
   a. Exercise
3. Have a health team and support group
   a. Functional Doctor
   b. Stress
   c. Acupuncture
      i. Yoga
      ii. Therapist
      iii. Dietitian
4. Make sleep a priority
5. Take Supplements with the guidance of a healthcare professional
   a. Multivitamin
   b. Omega 3
   c. Nootropics (Brain and Memory Supplements)
   d. Greens Drink Mix and Juice

PART 2

Regenerative Agriculture

The food system has displayed a movement towards unsustainability and scarcity in many respects.

The degradation of natural habitat and negative environmental impacts are significant. As is the continued decline in health across the world, Wade Lightheart (Podcast Number Three) pointed out that many of our health problems stem from a change in agriculture practices post WWII.

Again, I am not here to condemn what has happened, and I don't believe farmers have intentionally done anything to hurt the population. I think well-intentioned practices to make a living and provide food, sometimes have had unintended consequences.

While the health of Americans in particular is alarming, the root of the crisis began with food. Not just the food we eat but the way the food is grown. The amazing aspect of this all is by improving the system of agriculture, we can solve multiple issues that we face.

Dr. Allen Williams

Dr. Allen Williams is a champion of the grass-fed beef industry and an expert in grazing methodology and regenerative agriculture. He is a 6th generation farmer and founding partner of Grass Fed Beef LLC, and Grass Fed Insights LLC. He serves on the board for Grassfed Exchange and has written articles for *Graze*, *The Stockman Grassfarmer* and other publications. Williams has consulted with thousands of farmers and ranchers throughout the U.S., Canada, Mexico and South America. He is a partner in Joyce Farms, Inc.

Podcast Transcript Number: Dr. Allen Williams – World Renowned Regenerative Agriculture Expert

Logan: We are here with Dr. Allen Williams. World-renowned regenerative agriculture expert. Thank you so much for joining us and helping share some of the knowledge that you have.

Williams: Very good to be here. I really appreciate the opportunity.

Logan: Awesome. So we are in Arkansas, central Arkansas, and we shoot a lot of videos and work with farmers. And one of our missions honestly, it's to create a Blue Zone in Arkansas. So that's just an area around the world where people live to 100, a high-quality life. So if we can do it in one of the unhealthiest states in America, we can do it anywhere.

Williams: I agree with that.

Logan: So, researching all of this, my little boy was diagnosed with cancer in 2019. So stage four kidney cancer, and so we had our lives turned upside down. And so in researching, what do we do, how do I help him, and things like that. It's a rabbit trail, rabbit trail, to farming. It is so unbelievably important. So we feel like the way to make people healthier also solves a whole lot of problems with soil. So can you break down just the basic fundamental difference between conventional farming and regenerative agriculture?

Williams: Yeah, absolutely. In conventional farming, we rely very heavily on a lot of tools, technologies, and inputs, chemical inputs, synthetic inputs, things like that that frankly can be highly destructive. And not just destructive to the soil, but destructive to our environment, to our ecosystems, and also destructive to our health because we are significantly impacting nutrient density in the foods that we're consuming. However, with regenerative agriculture, what we're really doing is we're working with nature rather than against nature and pretty much every other type of agriculture that we try to do, we find ourselves always fighting against nature. Believe it or not, I actually hear farmers all the time talking about fighting against nature as if they're proud of it and somehow I'm going to beat nature. But I have a quote that I use quite often and it goes like this, "Nature will humble you. And if you refuse to be humbled, nature will beat you."

So starting with regenerative agriculture, what we're doing again is we're trying to implement agricultural practices and systems that allow us to work with nature and to be able to repair, restore, rebuild, and revitalize the four ecosystem processes. And that is the energy cycle, sunlight and photosynthesis, the water cycle, the mineral cycle, and what we call community dynamics or in essence, the diversity out here in the biological community, in these ecosystems. And to do that within regenerative agriculture, we use two primary things. We use the six principles of soil health and what we call the three rules of adaptive stewardship.

And so with that, when you're talking about these rules and stuff, you have a company, a consulting business with some amazing, amazing people, but you teach these principles. So you go out to a farm, that's been practicing it across the world, I guess. It's definitely across the United States, and teaches classes in which you can have other farmers come in. What is the most eye opening thing a lot of farmers see out of the gate?

The most eye opening thing quite frankly is the fact that they can actually implement regenerative practices and not lose money in the early years, because most of them think that this is more like the transition to certified organic. In the first three to five years, they're going to experience some kind of significant revenue loss, but with regenerative agriculture, that's just simply not the case. If you do this properly from year one, you can actually anticipate input cost reduction and revenue increases even in year one. So, that's probably the most eye opening thing. And I would say the second most eye-opening thing is the fact that they are entering into discovery and in that discovery what they're figuring out is that every day is a new day. They're seeing more immortal life exploding on their farms and anybody that's a farmer and rancher, that's pretty important to them.

Logan: That's a really interesting side effect in a positive way of applying regenerative practice. So we were recently out at one of my friends, the Ralstons farm, and they have a rice operation in which they have their own mill and they are implementing so many different practices. They don't necessarily have livestock running over where the rice fields were, but they're using a lot of surface runoff. They're doing the no till and they're not bailing the straw, so doing different things. So when we were out there, we saw beavers in the irrigation ditches, healthy, Bald Eagles, all kinds of birds. And so it's really cool to see they're working with nature. And so back to your point, we're not supposed to be fighting nature in the chemists, I guess, approach. It's more of a biology approach that we can be profitable, give back to nature, create habitat, and just win on every level.

Williams: Yeah. And that's a very good point because what has happened and I spent 15 years in academia as a research scientist. And clearly what I saw during that time period was that in spite of us coming up with all of these new technologies, and new products, and new methodologies, we were steadily seeing not only an erosion in farm net profit, net revenue, but we were also seeing a steady erosion in our soil health and our ecosystem health and our animal health and in just the overall populations of beneficial insects, birds, things like that. And so the bottom line really is what we're doing is we truly are restoring life and there's nothing more gratifying. That's why when we talk about the three rules, we call those the rules of adaptive stewardship. And we take that word stewardship quite seriously.

Logan:Yeah.

Williams: And it's really very heartening and heartwarming that we can begin to restore things much closer to the original state. And instead of seeing the degradation around us. For the last 80 years in our agricultural science, what we have done is we have assumed that the soil is all about chemistry and we have completely ignored biology. And that's now what, through regenerative agriculture, we are rediscovering that biology is really the driver. So for the past eight decades, we've acted as if chemistry drives biology, but it's actually the other way around. Biology drives chemistry. And when we get that right, everything starts to function a whole lot better.

Logan: It's really remarkable to me, the principles that are underlying life are across the board. So for what we've done up, recently you did an interview with Wade T. Lockhart, who was a Canadian bodybuilder. He owns a bio optimizer. He's fantastic. And he broke down exactly what you said, post-World War II, we started using chemical fertilizers and everything. It just kind of went to pot after that. The soil microbiome and the gut microbiome are so unbelievably similar in every way. We need a healthy soil microbiome. We need a good gut microbiome and a lot of the same approaches. So the pesticides, the herbicides, the glycol, you name it, it's the same thing. So we can really make a major impact on the health of humans and livestock by applying these principles.

Williams: That's absolutely correct and we teach that in our soil health academies, that the microbiome is the microbiome. And what we mean by that is that the microbiome in the soil should be strikingly similar to the microbiome in plants, in animals, in our livestock, and in us. And it's only when we alter that microbiome and it is different between our gut and the soil or the gut of our livestock and the soil that we then start to have problems. And those problems become compounding and cascading in effect and very negatively so. So you are absolutely correct. We've got to restore this original microbiome that has those incredible similarities between all living organisms.

Logan: Well, I love it. It's something that we can attack and do to make a major, major improvement. So something else that we've come across, I'd like for you to elaborate on, is that it seems that we are dealing with more droughts and more floods going on. Why is it that you believe soil is the solution to both of those?

Williams: That's a very good question. And just keeping in mind that we have worked throughout all of North America and with many other countries of the world. So to date, we've worked with 54 countries and counting and in every conceivable environment that you can think about, so everywhere from cold northern climates to hot humid climates, like what I live in down here in the deep South, to very arid, desert climates, and what we have found very clearly is that because of our poor agricultural practices and keeping soil exposed for so long out of the year, we have totally changed the dynamics of our climate because soil temperature has a ton to do with this. So it's not just the release of carbon and other greenhouse gases from the soil. Yes, that plays a major role in bare soil and constant tillage of that soil or frequent tillage certainly continuously releases those into the atmosphere. But it's also the temperature and the moisture holding capacity of the soil that is greatly contributing to our climate abnormalities and extremes.

And for instance, right here, where I am in Alabama, I'm at our farm here at BDA farm in Alabama today, and we have had in the month of

March, on the last day of March, and we have had a little better than 20 inches of rain in a single month. And we had another deluge of rain today and I drove into town and driving back, I was very disheartened because there was water running everywhere. This water unfortunately was not clear. It was very muddy. So all of these plowed fields that we have around here right now with this 20 plus inches of rain, they're losing nutrients, they're losing sediment, they're losing topsoil. So this is significantly damaging the ability of our client to function properly. And that is directly leading to more volatility in our weather, more severity in our weather, and obviously more flooding and more droughts.

One of the things that we've noted very definitively for instance, down in the Chihuahuan desert in Mexico at the Los Thomas ranch, one of the ranches that we've worked very heavily with in restoring regenerative practices, and that ranch is about 30,000 acres. We have found that on just a 30,000 acre landscape, just by re-greening that landscape through regenerative practices in the desert, we have created a microclimate on that ranch. And that ranch is now getting precipitation that the neighboring ranches do not get. And we have the radar evidence for year after year to back that up as well as the actual precipitation evidence. So we now know for a fact that if we implement the right practices, we can very favorably alter our climate and our environment.

Logan: That's really cool. So, the solution for both extremes, it goes back to the soil. So that analogy and correct me if I'm using the wrong analogy. What I tried to explain is that we want our soil to be very similar to a kitchen sponge. We want it to be able to soak up the water as much as possible, and then it will dissipate. We don't want it to be like a plate where it hits and then runs off. Right?

Williams: Yes.

Logan: And what that enables is for there not to be as extreme of flash floods for one, it doesn't get rid of a lot of the nutrients or organic material quickly. So it's just, all in all, keeping the ground cover is a big deal, isn't it? And keeping those living roots.

Williams: It is a huge deal.

Logan: Why is that hard to get, or why is that hard to embrace?

Williams: That's a very good question. And we get asked the question all the time, "Well, if regenerative agriculture is so great, why isn't everybody doing it?" And actually, oftentimes I like to say, well, "there's never a dumb question, but I'm going to make the exception now and say, that's actually a dumb question because no matter how good something is, not everybody does it, right?"

Logan: So if drinking to excess is bad for you, but we still have people that do it.

Williams: Yeah. Right.

Drugs to excess is bad for you, but we still have people that do it. So 100% are never going to adopt anything. That's just people in life. But the fact of the matter is that you cannot implement what you do not know and the vast majority of farmers and ranchers out there still today do not understand regenerative agriculture. They do not understand those six principles and those three rules of adaptive stewardship that I talked about earlier. And so education is the very first step to helping them begin to understand how to implement the principles and rules on their farms.

Logan: And so I've watched the amazing mini documentaries that you've done with the carbon cowboy and the Mark Hyman podcast is something I think everybody should go out and listen to. I think that was just phenomenal. I've listened to it at least seven times, but after listening to your stuff, one of the biggest things that I go back to is, I'm from a rural community, a small town. It's like 2000 people and I can just remember, everybody had cattle. The cattle were on the same pasture 100% of the time. They would have summer where they ate the grass, winter they supplemented all year and they put in hay. And I can hear some of these older farmers saying, "But it's wasted pasture. If I don't have something on it, it's wasted." So, what is your way of addressing that?

Williams: So, number one, you're exactly right. Unfortunately, that's the way that the majority of grazers graze and not just here in the U.S. but globally. And just like the majority of farmers in the U. S. and globally do excess tillage and apply too many synthetics and chemicals. The way that we do it though, we call it biomimicry and ecomimicry. So we use a grazing methodology that we developed called adaptive grazing. The vast majority of grazers basically follow a prescriptive or formulaic type of grazing, where they do the same thing all the time, day in and day out, year in and year out. And that just simply does not work. It is going to degrade the soil and the ecosystem. No doubt about it. But with adaptive grazing, what we're doing is we're trying to mimic the wild ruminants, the vast herds of wild ruminants that once existed and roamed the face of this earth and in a North America, that would have been the bison, the antelope, and all of that.

And so we mimic their patterns the way they moved across the landscape. They never stayed.

Logan: They weren't fenced in somewhere.

Williams: Not at all. They were moving every single day. And so that's what we do too. We move every day. So, we use temporary fencing technology or herding. And both work very well, depending on the size and ruggedness of the landscape. And we literally move our livestock to a fresh bite of grass every single day. Now, just that one simple thing, now there's more to it than that, but if that's all you did, if you just simply moved them to a fresh paddock every single day, we are immediately growing a lot more grass. We're immediately creating a lot more soil biology and diversity in the plant species, and beneficial insects, birds, and so forth. And we are immediately restoring water infiltration rates, soil aggregation, and all of these other things that are so vital to a healthy soil.

Logan: So by growing grass, what we see, they're also growing roots that are adding more organic material and doing a lot more things that you can dive into with biology. So it's both ways. It's up and down. It's more feed. It's more biodiversity but it's also adding bulk and those roots die. They add organic material and now we create that sponge, a better sponge. Okay. So when you're saying that, I go back to the discovery channel and they're over in Africa and then millions of Wildebeest are out just roaming. They're just moving over a huge, huge area and they may not see that ground again for months, if not a year, right?

Williams: Yep. Yep. I'm sorry. I lost you there for that last statement.

Logan: So the Wildebeest just moving on, they may not come across the same ground again for up to a year.

Williams: That's correct. And what we have found is that every grassland needs rest. And when we allow that rest, then we are going to have degradation in the soil, in the plant species' diversity, and in all of the other diversity that exists there. So those rest periods are critical and just simply by grouping your animals up and moving them as I described earlier, day by day, across that landscape, you totally change the dynamics.

Everything changes for the better. And the biggest drawback we hear initially before anybody actually does this, "Oh my gosh, that's going to take way too much time. I can't move my cows every day. I can't move my sheep every day." Or, "I can't move my chickens every day." But the truth is absolutely, yes you can. And it takes far less time than you think and what you really doing is your exchange in labor for labor, because if I don't move them every day, I've got to spend a lot of time in the summertime cutting, raking, baling, and putting up hay to feed them through the winter. And then I've got to spend a lot of time in the winter feeding all that hay back as well as buying other expensive feed supplements to maintain them during the week. So all you're really doing is just exchanging labor for labor. And yet just through that one to one exchange, we're getting significantly more positive benefits and results.

Logan: That's awesome. Also breaking a lot of the fly cycles. You get healthier animals and less in vet bills, supplements, and stuff. All right. I want to take us in a little bit different direction because I think it's extremely important. I own a farmer's market. So I've worked directly with lots and lots of farmers and something that has just come to my attention is kind of twofold. One, a lot of them aren't making money. And so we've got to figure out what we can do. And so from the retail side, I'm trying to spend a lot of time on that and how we help and have more of an outlet and more people appreciating local products or higher quality. The other thing is I didn't realize how depression and suicide is running rampant for a lot of farmers. I had no idea. What can we do now and long-term to help with that?

Williams: That is exactly correct and that's exactly what we have found that farmer depression and farmer suicide rates, both here in the U.S. and many other countries around the world have exploded. And that has created just a significant problem with families, quality of life, everything else that we're now dealing with. And a lot of that is due to the fact that as I mentioned earlier, farm profits have eroded dramatically. And so what we find with regenerative agriculture, and this is one of the things that make what we do on a daily basis so really good is that we see lives restored, not just soil restored, and land restored, and ecosystems restored, but we see lives restored, families restored because when they start in to regenerative agriculture, this helps them break the debt cycle that they're under. The crushing load of debt that many of these farm families have been enduring.

So they're able to break the debt cycle, get out from under their debt and they're able to start enjoying a much higher quality of life. And the thing that they tell us over and over again is that this has been the most freeing experience of my life. And I could give you many examples. I'm going to give you one, but Adam Grati who farms in Eastern North Carolina near Kenansville, he's a 10th generation farmer. So the land's been in their family since the 1780s. They were over the last decade or so, they've been really struggling and it was getting tougher and tougher for them. And when you think about that heritage, since the 1780s, 10th generation and Adam's sitting here thinking, "Oh my gosh, am I going to be the generation to lose the farm?"

So enormous pressure on him. And he was introduced to regenerative agriculture in the fall of 2016. They started implementing it that fall. And by 2018, on 1200 acres, just his second year in, Adam had saved $200,000 in input cost, $200,000. By the end of the third year, Adam called me up the week after Thanksgiving and said, "Allen, I'm just returning from my bank. I just met with my lender and I just paid off all my loans." He said, "I'm debt-free." And he said, "Oh, by the way, I just bought another farm paying all cash for it."

Logan: Love it.

Williams: And in 2020, Adam acquired yet another farm. So just-

Logan: That's awesome.

Williams: When you hear that in the people that we've been able to be a part of their lives and they have achieved that because of what we've been able to teach them, it's very uplifting and it keeps us doing what we're doing.

Logan: I love it. I love it. So anything that is going to help as many problems for the solutions, I can get behind. So I think this is a big deal. I want to be able to help bring the knowledge you all have to Arkansas.

So we definitely want to stay in contact with you all and see where you can do an event here and have you speak and just share your wisdom and practices, because I think it's a big, big deal. And is there a preferred means that you want people to come find out more about you, a website or email, Facebook, where do people need to come find you?

Williams: Absolutely, so there's three websites that they can visit us at. They can visit us at understandingag.com. They can visit us at thesoilhealthacademy.org and at bdafarm.com. And so we welcome anybody to visit there, and if they want to contact me directly, they can do so by emailing me at Allen, A-L-L-E-N @understandingag.com.

Logan: Allen, thank you so much for the time. And what you're doing is making a huge difference for our country and everybody that applies it. So thank you, thank you, thank you.

Regenerative agriculture is a holistic approach that positively affects a wide range of issues.

- Human Health
- Livestock
- Wildlife
- Soil health
- Soil conservation
- Water conservation
- Biodiversity
- Soil Carbon Cycle

Regenerative Agriculture and Regenerative Health both focus on improving ecosystem health.

The resilience of farms shows up in many ways, one extremely important is increased profitability.

Ralston Family Farms:

I'm from a small town called Atkins, Arkansas, located about halfway between Little Rock and Fort Smith along the Arkansas River.

For a long time our little community was dependent upon the pickle plant. As the primary employer, the pickle plant bought locally grown cucumbers from around the area creating a product they distributed across the country.

After a few decades, the pickle plant was transferred, costing a significant number of jobs and many farmers lost their primary outlet for the crops they grew. The negative impacts had a ripple effect that has lasted for a long time, even to the point where the annual pickle festival has become more of a sleepwalk, than a new invigorating event.

A few years back Tim and Robin Ralston, who are River Valley farmers, put in a rice mill to package for retail the rice they grew in their farming operation.

What I love about what the Ralstons are doing is that they are utilizing Regenerative Agriculture for their rice mill operation. They are cognizant that it is good for the environment, while allowing them to have a profitable business.

The Ralstons have worked with a myriad of different agencies in order to do things to the best of their ability.

One aspect I find extremely interesting is the fact that they are part of a water irrigation group. Those types of boards can be set up in different ways, but for the one in the Atkins area, they pull from the Arkansas River irrigation canals and pump it onto their zero grade rice fields. What is fascinating about this method is they pull in the dirty, muddy water from the river, and by the time it leaves the fields or leeches into the ground, it is crystal clear. The vegetation acts as filters, like a natural wetland.

We filmed an episode of the TV show, Good Roots, on PBS at the Ralston's Farm. There we witnessed fields teeming with abundant wildlife. From Bald Eagles and beavers, to a ton of different bird species, life in this area was thriving.

The future is bright for the Ralstons, and I can see how Atkins, Arkansas could become an agricultural hub with rice as a central product.

Action Step

1. Shop at Farmer's Markets and/or buy directly from farmers
   a. Support farmers using Regenerative Farming practices
   b. Encourage farmers to adopt Regenerative Agriculture methods
      i. Rotational Grazing
      ii. No till, covercrops
      iii. Silvopasture
      iv. Permaculture

PART 3

Regenerative Business

Regenerative Business is a concept that I am incredibly passionate about. In that, it is a business that gives back to the community to provide positive growth, with positive results. For me, the fundamental ways in which we can benefit the community is by providing goods and services that contribute to health and prosperity.

The other side of providing goods and service, however, is that the business still needs to be profitable and provide for the owner's financial freedom. I believe through the creation of business - more opportunities are therefore created.

Be not deceived; God is not mocked: for whatsoever a man soweth, that shall he also reap. Galatians 6:7, KJV

Dave Asprey, the founder of Bulletproof is a hero and role model of mine. His work has changed the lives of countless lives and I've referred to his work many times in this book. The majority of supplements and experts I've learned from originated from Dave. He has been able to create an extraordinary business which is positively impacting the world. This concept fully embodies the regenerative business I'm outlining.

I've seen firsthand the positive impact, Me & McGee Market, a little produce stand can have on a community.

However, in a money-first economy, greed and self-servingness often lead motivation.

Therefore, to support all of the audacious goals of implementing and developing Regenerative Businesses, we must have successful businesses connecting back to the prosperity theme - Sowing Prosperity.

For the movement and implementation of regenerative initiatives across healthcare, grocery, food services, and agriculture, businesses must be set up to succeed. There are a ton of books on success, and I've been blessed to have had a burning desire to learn the business.

I've seen statistics of business failure all over the place. It's widely evident most new businesses fail. Forbes has reported up to 90%.

It doesn't matter what business we are in, we focus on the agriculturally-related businesses that have common principles for success.

Capitalism

I want to hit on something that at one time I struggled with growing up. I heard over and over, "Money is the root of all evil."

I've gone over this concept a lot more with one of my early mentors, Tony Moore. I think it's essential to state here that if one believes money is evil, then capitalism in its entirety, by that definition is then evil. This cannot be further from reality.

Capitalism has gotten a bad name in many respects, for a good reason. Back to the Bible verse first in which reading the full verse is extremely important:

1 Timothy 6:10 KJV

For the love of money is the root of all evil: which while some coveted after, they have erred from the faith, and pierced themselves through with many sorrows.

This is much different than money is evil. Money is no more than a means of exchange in which societies can utilize.

All of this is extremely important as the first layer of a successful business, especially for many farmers who feel guilty about making money.

Money is not bad. It is simply a medium of exchange. Creating a profitable business is one of the best ways to strengthen a community.

Whole Foods founder John Mackey has a fantastic book, *Conscious Capitalism*, and I encourage everyone to read it.

In the book, John refers to a cooperative produce farmer's market in which the bureaucracy makes decisions too slowly. In speaking to a farmer about his experience with a cooperative, he echoed the slow decision-making. He was stuck with an abundance of produce when they ultimately went out of business.

"It's capitalism that creates innovations that create the progress in the world and it's lifting humanity literally out of the dirt."

I have seen the impact of bringing together quality farmers, food service, and retail, in terms of a stronger system that provides value to everyone, including the consumer.

I want to highlight an example of how Me & McGee Market has used this model to make positive meat changes.

Hoien Family Farms is a grass-fed beef operation in my hometown of Atkins, Arkansas. They are a great small business and family. They genuinely care about the land, the cattle, and the consumers of their meat.

By partnering with us at Me & McGee, we buy a significant amount of their meat. We do this for the reasons as mentioned earlier. They care for their land and use rotational grazing techniques that are massively beneficial for their farm and the environment, as per the conversation and work of Dr. Allen Williams.

Also, by raising their cattle on healthy diverse grassland, the cattle are healthier. These healthier cattle have more nutritious meat for higher vitamin, mineral, and Omega 3 fatty acids.

The healthier meat is sold at our market and used on our food truck by Chef Josh Smith, The Southern Standard. Using the meat on the food truck, we can showcase the high-quality meat and sell more. When we sell more, we buy more. This strengthens and benefits everyone involved while motivating the continued use of regenerative farming practices.

If farmers are unable to make a living, we will lose even more of them.

Many times, niche farmers are unable to have profitable businesses. This, many times, is because they don't look at what they do as a business.

Early Mentor Tony Moore:

I can't stress enough that a profitable business is a good thing. Those principles are something that makes the difference between an impactful enterprise and a soul-draining experience.

Profitable businesses are able to buy more inventory, hire more employees, reinvest in the business and better provide a service to others.

I visited with one of my early mentors, who has achieved great success in the real estate industry and investor.

I am here with one of the very early mentors who, honestly, I didn't fully appreciate at the time, but looking back, I used something Tony said just about every single day in business.

Podcast Transcript: Tony Moore, Real Estate Broker, Investor and Arkansas Real Estate Commissioner

Logan: So, I am with Tony Moore, real estate legend here in Arkansas, Arkansas Real Estate Commission, and owner of many offices scattered up and down the River Valley. Very glad to have him.

Tony, I want to hit on something. We're talking about farmers and agriculture and business on how they can be profitable. One thing that you drilled in my head, and every other real estate agent, was to make the main thing, the main thing. Why is that important? And why is that something that you have used over these years?

Tony: Well, it's easy, Logan; get your eye on the most critical ball for business. People have great concepts; they have a good product. They have thought through niche marketing; maybe they have a good, solid customer base. Often, they don't understand their expenses and what it costs to provide a product, and they don't know the full cost of all the aspects of it. So they're not profitable and they will be under-capitalized almost every time. In small business, the number one reason it fails is under-capitalization. They lose their cash in little bitty places where they don't realize that they're not making money. They're actually losing money, but it's in small bites, and so all of a sudden, their cash flow evaporates and there is nothing to substantiate the business growth so they go borrow money. And that cycle then gets larger, more ominous and it ends up [inaudible 00:02:01].

The main thing on the main thing is trying to... The head of Murphy Oil, once upon a time, was at a family meeting, so Murphy is Murphy USA and its Deltic Timber, and he said to his kids," put all your eggs in one basket and take extremely great care of that basket." So the 70's come along, the 80's come along and they started by diversify, diversify, diversify, killed so many businesses because maybe they would be really good at this and maybe fair at that, but really poor at this and that, that they were really poor, just sucked all their cash down. So focus; keep the main thing, the main thing. For the application is that is to farming and forth is that diversification can kill you if not able to manage; you can diversify and lots of different things that you don't know what you're doing and lose your rear end.

So, focus, keep the main thing, the main thing. For me, I am in the real estate business, this is what I do 12 to 14 hours a day. I focus on it. I want to be the best at it. And I never get my eye off of it. I'm not going to do anything else, but this right here, and I'm going to be the very best at what I'm doing. And I'm going to be able to make the profits because I know this business. So focus, just keep the main thing, the main thing is bear down, double down, and then go to work.

Logan: I love it. So, when I became a partner in Me and McGee market, one of the first things that I really brought to the table was," we can do anything, but we can't do everything." So, we had to figure out how we got back to the main thing. What was the main thing? And stay focused on it. With that, something else you used to say all the time was, " it's not the elephants that'll get you, it's the mosquitoes." What do you mean by that?

Tony: So, for you Logan and your enterprise that you're dealing with now, if you manage pennies, dollars will take care of themselves. The best managers are managing based on the principle of," watch the little details." You don't have to be a micromanager now, but getting back to basics... There's a guy there on the wall, Vince Lombardi, started every football season with a bunch of pros saying, " this is a football;

it is measured by yards, and won by inches. It is won by fundamentals and businessmen [inaudible 00:05:01], so it's about your Facebook, your computerization, this, that. No it's not, it's about product, cost management and customer service. Those are the main... he said," well, that's not very exciting, that's not very cutting edge. Goodness gracious. Should we improve? We need to improve our website. No, maybe you need to improve your counter, voice inflection. Maybe we need to talk about how we're interfacing with customers, taking care of people, because as we get more and more disenfranchised from dealing face-to-face with people who becomes more and more important because people are going to go backwards to say," I miss interaction, I miss customer service."

Logan: We're seeing that every day.

Tony: They truly want shopping, buying, experiencing, or seeing people. They want to hear about [inaudible 00:06:02]. So, forget the darn website. Is it important? Yeah, but it's not as important as how you deal with people.

Logan: I think we've gotten so far away from Dale Carnegie teachings and it just is evident in every form of business. A lot of the farmer's markets and stuff that I've seen: you go by and they're laying back, they've got their vegetables set up there, but they're laying back reading the paper, they're no more interested in having a conversation with somebody that comes up. When you don't make people feel important, you're not going to earn their business.

Tony: Amazon's going to take your business from you. So the elephants don't bite, but mosquitoes get you. If you're not watching a small business today, the elephant, the 800 pound gorilla is Amazon. And if you don't provide that customer an outstanding experience into step out of the wallpaper, because you're never going to be able to beat him on price now.

Logan: Ever.

Tony: And so if you don't think that elephant's not going to get you, so the mosquito is: take care and provide a great experience; help your customer; love on them; treat them like royalty, or the elephant that's in the other room, that 800 pound gorilla they're going to go down and sit on her laptop out in the car on the phone and order it. And it'd be sitting at your doorstep in 24 hours and you're whooped.

Logan: So, this is very much in line with something else that you said regularly," if you want to be average, do what the average do." That's something that stayed with me, and so I look more in business at ourselves more than I even do it as quote, unquote, "competition." I want to be the best at whatever it is that I'm doing; I want to be better today than I was yesterday, and I want to look at how I improve for tomorrow. The average I feel in our industries, and this is why it's so important on this topic, they try to do exactly what the other markets are doing or the other farms. They want to grow the same type of okra or squash or tomatoes. They want to have the exact same thing. And then that creates average across the board instead of being special and being known as one thing. So do you have any example of exceptional that comes to mind?

Tony: So, picture a track meet me and you're setting up in the stands and it's the two-mile-long race, and there's 20 people going to be running this race. And so that's about what eight laps, I think. So within that, they all start out in one great big bunch, but after about the second lap, all of a sudden, watch what happens in almost every two-mile race, there'll be two or three that start pulling away from the rest of the pack. And as they go around one more time, watch what happens: the two or three lead begins to be greater and the pack remains the same. Now which one is, it is a two or three running that much faster than the 12 or is the 12 slowing down so they can stay together because there's comfort in the pack. So I submit to you, it could be some of both, but a lot of times it's the comfort of running shoulder to shoulder in a pack of mediocrity.

Logan: Here we go again, another "Tonyism" a very eye opening way of elaborating that.

Tony: So, in business, we began to look across the aisle at what somebody else is doing, as long as I match that level of excellence is always peaked at whatever it takes to be equal to him. So it stops our creativity, our growth, our progression in trying to look at other avenues and do things different, innovative, we become complacent. And so it's easy to say because I'm at least equal with him and why not be authentic and be out in the front?

So many knowledge bombs right there.

(Laughs).

Logan: Just wisdom. I miss this Tony, I really do. All right. One more thing that I feel is extremely important, especially with a lot of the farmers that I work with directly: a lot of times I almost had a guilty feeling towards making money; a guilty feeling towards charging for growing healthy food that will benefit other people. So with that, a lot of times that we hear quoted is the Bible. And what I hear typically is different than what the scripture actually says. So, if you can elaborate on that. If I hear, "money is the root of all evil" and that is not exactly what the Bible verse says and that is " the love of money is the root of all evil which while some coveted after they are erred from the faith and pierced themselves through with many sorrows". You are a very respected man of God, especially in my book, and I would like your take on that...

Tony: Well, thank you for that, Logan, that's very kind of you. But, it's the love of money is the root of all kinds of evil. Money is ethereal; it's nothing other than that phone on his desk. It's a medium or means of exchange. So in and of itself, it's an ethereal product; it has no good or bad in itself. It's not how much money I have, it's how much money has me that makes a difference. So, if you were to take the Bible verse, great verse, and say, " it's about the covetousness, about what is the desire of money and the show of money and all of those things, that's when money has you", but money in and of itself is... God has given us the opportunity and said, "put your hand to the plow and don't look back."

And if he's in it and a part of that triumph that is a blessing from him is the rewards of hard work and labor. Should it be hoarded up for our own selfish usage? No, it ought to be shared. He never gave it to us to pile it up, sit on top of it. He intends for us to put it at good utility, but it's his blessing and there's nothing wrong. Success, often is the greatest diminishing force to success. There are many people out there who think they want to be successful, but as they start becoming successful, that means we're pulling away from the pack. And they'd go back to the comfort of being in that pack. And that's true of every aspect of success and that's money. And so, that's God's blessing on digging what you do for a living.

And that's where enthusiasm is simply just "en theos", that means, "God within". I think it's digging what you're doing. And then he rewards you by giving you money as a blessing. So I've a fair profit. Look what he told Amos, he says," you've put gold in bags and I've cut holes in them because you've forgotten me." He says," if you will not do good, good is coming to you, I'll be good to you, just don't mistreat the widows and the orphans. Don't gouge people." He said," do not have an unholy balance on your scales. Don't you put false..." So they had scales to weigh out peanuts and they would create a one pound weight and they hollowed it out in the center so it was half a pound. So they were cheating people, Logan, of half a pound of peanuts. God says," I watch the scale."

Now it's good for the common, ordinary businessman, real state men, grocers or whoever it is to always remember God watches every scale of every balance. And he says, "don't you take advantage of poor people, don't you take advantage of people and I'll take care of your business." And I truly believe any business will prosper. And I do believe any business that's based on good moral sound things for people that looks to take care of customers, take care of people: God will take care of you if you take care of him, and that's true.

Logan: I'm with you Tony. Thank you so much.

Marketing

The approach I've taken to marketing at Me & McGee has been very different than anything I've seen.

I personally am tired of being "sold to" and don't want to sell to others. I want to relay information in a positive, informational and entertaining way.

Quality pictures are used as an enjoyable way to create a relationship with the audience, especially on social media.

The other way we market is indirectly through creating video content in an educational way.

For example, we went to Fox, Arkansas to visit a Bison Farm. The owner operator, Rod, is another great example of someone who cares for the land, animals and consumers. By going to the farm to film we were able to share the experience for many people who will never make it out. They learned and are even more a part of a product they can buy at Me & McGee Market.

Entrepreneurs are the true heroes in a free-enterprise economy, driving progress in business, society, and the world. They solve problems by creatively envisioning different ways the world could and should be.

Every person alive has the potential to learn and grow to contribute their unique creativity toward making the world a better place.

Podcast Transcript Number:

John Lee Dumas Award Winning Podcaster - Entrepreneurs on Fire

John Lee Dumas is the host of Entrepreneurs on Fire, an award-winning podcast where he interviews inspiring entrepreneurs who are truly ON

FIRE. With over 2500 episodes, 1 million listeners per month, and 7 figures of annual revenue. He is one of the trail blazers in the world of podcasting.

Much like Dave Asprey, John Lee Dumas or affectionately known as JLD to Fire Nation is a major influence on my life leading me to many of the experts I've learned from in business and life. Including my business coach Clay Clark.

John: Logan!

Logan: What are you doing, buddy?

John: You know, Puerto Rico's exciting, our birds are singing. Life is good.

Can it get any better?

Logan: I love it. Well, I've made it through your book on audible about four times now.

John: What?

Logan: So I've got all the hard copies in. I got 50 of them.

John: I got a question for you.

Logan: Yeah.

John: Have you left me a kind review yet?

Logan: It's happening today. As soon as we wrap this up, it's done.

John: I believe you.

Logan: Alright, brother. I know you got other things to do, so I appreciate you taking the time to do this.

Just a tiny bit of background on us. I've got a farmer's market in Arkansas. So, middle of Arkansas, in Little Rock. My little boy was diagnosed with cancer, 2019, stage four. And so we just embraced health and embraced that journey. And so in doing that, my goal is to create a Blue Zone in Arkansas. So, if we can take one of the unhealthiest states in the country and create a Blue Zone, we've accomplished a lot and got rid of a lot of the negatives.

So with that, you have had a ton of success, even spending time with Tony Robbins on his private island. So that's pretty cool. What are your thoughts about the correlation between health and success?

John: It's everything. And I mean, 100% everything. There's a quote that I love that says, "The person with health wants 10,000 things. The person without health wants one thing." They want their health.

Logan: That's beautiful.

John: Nothing matters, Logan, without the health. Literally nothing matters. And I'm actually speaking from experience, like I'm on the tail end, right now, of COVID. I've had it now for about two weeks-

Logan: Oh, man!

John: it put me out of commission for a couple of days. And I've been on the slow mend ever since. And I'll tell you, man, when you're down and out with something like that, nothing else matters except getting better.

Logan: Absolutely. So even with the COVID, that's obviously something I didn't know that you were dealing with. But you embrace a very healthy lifestyle. So what do you eat to prepare for that? And what did you notice with COVID specifically?

John: Yeah, so I'm very committed to eating healthy, to taking daily supplements, to taking my daily nutritional support powder and fruits and vegetables. And I'm always committed to that. I eat very little meat, mostly vegetables. I'm just always committed to putting the right things in my body.

In fact, there's a fantastic book, I highly recommend for anybody that's listening right now, called *The Pleasure Trap*. And it really helps us understand how food has trapped us over the years. And people in Arkansas, like you said, being one of the more unhealthy states, it's because they're trapped by the pleasure trap. And it's really an addictive drug, this thing called food, and sugar, and everything that goes along with that. And getting out of that is just so difficult because it is like breaking an addiction.

And in fact, I'm going to a wellness center where I'm going to be doing a 10-day water-only fast.

Logan: Wow.

John: Really allow my body to completely just flush out, clean out, reset. I don't know how much you've gone into details about learning about autophagy and things along those lines. And I'm really excited about it. In fact, the author of this book runs this center called The True North Health Center up in Santa Rosa, California.

I will definitely check that out. Now, Valter Longo, longevity expert, he's big into fasting, and fasting-mimicking diet. And autophagy's a big deal in combating cancer, which is -

John: Big time.

Logan: ...one of our big, big passions. So you live in Puerto Rico ... you're originally from Maine, right?

John: Yep.

Logan: And then moved down to Puerto Rico. Do y'all have farmer's markets down there?

John: So we do have farmer's markets down here. You know, Puerto Rico is a thriving agricultural island. 'Cause the weather is year-round, you can really get three harvests a year here. I actually have my own organic garden in my yard here where I have greens, vegetables, all the tomatoes. I have a fruit orchard of mangoes, papayas, lemons, and plantains. So, I'm all about just going outside and harvesting the food that I have planted and grown right outside of it.

Logan: It tastes so much better when it just goes from the yard to the house.

John: So much better.

Logan: So much better. So with the Regenerative Agriculture and health and things, I'm very passionate about helping the farmers or those in that industry be successful. We've been very blessed at Me and McGee Market and what we've done, but a big part of that is the food chain, and just being able to market and do things. What have you noticed? Maybe going down to a farmer's market where there's a vendor or something that stands out, that they may be doing, that you can share?

John: So, when I like to visit farmer's markets, I like to go and ask what the story is. I think the story is fascinating. So, when I go to farmer's markets and when I see people that are doing things differently, those are the people that are willing to come out from behind the counter and tell a story. Tell the story [inaudible 00:06:03] of what is the reason why they're growing that specific product. Like what is the reason why, this is the thing that they're coming to the farmer's market for? Like what is the family history? Like why is this something that they are essentially spending their lives doing, because how we spend our days is how we spend our lives. And I love the story.

So whenever I'm at farmer's markets, I'm always asking for the background, I'm always asking for the details and some people don't want to talk about it, and I get it, and that's their prerogative. But the ones that I really see doing some special things are people that really jump on the opportunity to tell their story because it's fascinating.

Logan: I love that. And that story is big, and being open and honest, you build up relationships. I picked that up in some of your early mentors, like I believe it was Jamie that you felt like you knew her because you had listened to her story when y'all first met, even though you hadn't met. But-

John:...that's really neat, the story.

Logan: With your book, *The Common Path to Uncommon Success*, it wasn't necessarily geared towards agriculture or anything, but I feel there's a lot of principles in there that can apply. Well, some of the things that stood out for me were creating an avatar, focus, that's a big one for farmers. Okay? 'Cause they want to do everything. Focus, niches and masterminds. That's all in your book. And that's one of the biggest reasons I want to make sure that I can get it out to them. But can you expand on where you can see that correlation? And why are those things so important?

John: Listen, those things are critical because if you don't have focus, you are not doing the one critical thing that over three thousand entrepreneurs that I've interviewed for this book have all done. They have followed one course until success. You know what would happen if you went and you planted a bunch of seeds and then the next day you just went and you picked them all up and you planted in some other seeds? That's what people do.

That's what people are doing over and over again. They're never giving their seeds an opportunity to bloom. You know, you've got to take time, you've got to water them, you've got to nurture them, you've got to focus on them. And then guess what? They will produce for you. But not if you're just going and planting and ripping them up and trying new, then and be like, why isn't this working? It's been 24 hours. It's been 48 hours. Like what's going on?

But that's what people do. I like to say they go one mile wide with all these different ideas and only one inch deep with their actual impact. And they wonder why they're not making any impact. It's the people, Logan, that go one inch wide and they go one mile deep. Those are the people that really commit to focusing, to following one course until success becomes the best, because guess what people want. People want the best solution to a real problem that they're having. And when you can provide the best solution to a real problem, people will beat a path to your doorstep because people want the best solution to their problem. And they will ignore the second best solution to infinity.

To make it personal for you for a second, if you found the second-best solution to your son's cancer, when he was four years old, and that person lived right next door, but you found the number one best solution, and it was halfway around the world. What would you do?

Logan: We're going around the world.

John: You're going around the world because that's what people want. They want the number one best solution to their problem. And even though that person's your next-door neighbor, and I'm sure they're great people and you love them, hey, the second best is not enough for your son who's struggling with cancer right now. Your son deserves and will get the best solution to a real problem he's having. And that is across the board, in everything in this world.

Logan: I love that. I love it … and agree wholeheartedly.

Something else to tie back into everything that we're doing: Mental health has been such a bigger focus, especially with the pandemic and the negatives. So with you being a wartime veteran, and you've been very open and honest with the PTSD that had to deal with and overcome, and thank you so much for going out and sacrificing for our country. Much, much, much appreciation.

John: Thank you, Logan.

Logan: But with that, what can we do to help, whether it's veterans or it is people that have just had a hard, hard time. Tie all of this together with nutrition and things. What have you found, JLD, to help?

John: So, number one when it comes to veterans, 22 veterans on average are committing suicide every single day because of PTSD. And I want to tell you what: It is a sad road that people get put down because people, they want the best for these veterans. They want the best for anybody. You know, these doctors they're doing what they can.

But what happened when I went to my doctor for PTSD? My doctor prescribed me pills, pharmaceutical pills. She never asked me what I was eating. She never asked me if I was eating sugar. She never asked me if I was drinking alcohol. She never asked me if I was doing drugs. Nothing. They just prescribed me pills. And so I just went back and I just kept eating the crap that I was eating back in the day. And it was a drain of despair where you keep going down, because food is a drug, food is addictive.

And if you're not putting the right foods in your body you are not going to be mentally sleeping that well, you know what I mean, mentally that clear. You're not going to be mentally that enthusiastic or excited to do the things you want to do because your health is everything. It allows you to wake up in the morning, excited to jump out of bed and tackle the day, as opposed to just lying in bed all day, just going down that further depths of despair.

And this might sound a little dramatic, for some people, not for you, Logan, 'cause you get it, but it might sound dramatic for some people. But believe me, it is not. 'Cause when you start giving your body the energy, and the nutrition, and the supplements, and the food that it needs to run. Now you're taking this unbelievably fine-tuned car that we are, this engine, and you're giving it the best ingredients. Opposed to, like you would never buy a Ferrari and then start just pouring castor oil into it.

But that's what we do with our bodies. Our bodies are Ferraris. They're unbelievable machines. Yet, the fuel that we put in our bodies is junk. And we wouldn't do that to our cars, but we do that to ourselves every single day.

It's just, we're so far away from the majority of people that need to know these things, from knowing them, that we still have a long way to go. I love what you're doing in your part of the woods, making Arkansas a Blue Zone, or at least your area in Arkansas, a Blue Zone. I think that's fantastic. And that's what we need. We need people like yourself and others. And hopefully at some point doctors, like the ones that I went to, to say, "Well, John, what did you eat today? Oh, you had fruit loops for breakfast, you had a pop tart for lunch, and then you had crap for dinner. No surprise you're not happy, and you're depressed. It's definitely due to some parts of your PTSD with your war, but let's get you on a healthy meal plan. Let's get you fasting. Let's get you exercising every day." That's what this world needs.

Logan: So that has made a big impact for you?

John: Everything.

Logan: Everything. So what I didn't realize. I just recently interviewed one of the top experts in Regenerative Agriculture, Dr. Alan Williams. And he let me know that farmers' suicide rates are at a ridiculous high.

John: Wow.

Logan: I didn't fully understand that. So the debt load they have, the commodity-farming prices. They don't make their own decisions, honestly, it is the farm insurance or it's grant money, or it's this, they're kind of dictated what they have to do. So they're not in control during life. You know, we're happy to the degree that we're in control of our own lives.

And so with that again, it's a lot of the similarities with the PTSD and the high stress load. So, most of them aren't healthy either. So I'm trying to create that awareness of, hey, let's focus on this regenerative, positive agricultural system. Let's focus on the regenerative health, the functional medicine, diet nutrition, and bring it all together. 'Cause we got a short time on this earth. We need to just really take care of each other and know how to get through it.

John: Can't agree with you more, brother. And especially, I'm sure once you start having kids, like you've had, you just have one son or do you have more?

Logan: I got four kids.

John: You know that, hey, they're going to have kids at some point, and those kids are going to have kids. And what kind of earth are we leaving them? That's something that needs to really start being thought about.

Logan: It is. All right. I know you got to get off here, buddy, but is there anything else you want to just let us know?

John: Honestly, let you know, thank you for what you do. I think it's incredibly important. And I think just you having the mentality of creating that Blue Zone where you live is an amazing start. If other people want to be inspired by the 3000 interviews that I've done over the past decade and the knowledge I've put into these 71,000 words, 273 pages, go check out uncommonsuccessbook.com, and you'll be on fire.

Logan: It's well worth it, and I'm headed to leave out reviews across all the platforms.

John: Yes. Logan-

Logan: JLD, thank you buddy.

EPILOGUE

I hope the book has been an eye-opening opportunity to know we have control over much of our lives.

My favorite Bible verse is Galatians 6:7:

Do not be deceived, God is not mocked; for whatever a man sows, that he will also reap.

Our lives are manifestations of seeds we've sown in the past and therefore the future is what seeds we sow in the present.

Regardless of what life throws our way, we can make the best of it by having faith in God, and focusing on the aspects we can control.

Lander has done exceedingly well, but has a lifetime of health focus. He is getting to be a little boy and currently is in the second grade. He has already been an influence in eating healthy and is a beacon of hope in desperate situations.

I'm honored to be his father and as difficult as the journey to this point has been, God has blessed the journey. Had it not been for cancer, life would look nothing like it does now.

Regenerative forms of agriculture, business, medicine and community will change the world for the better. I'm excited to be a part of it.

A brighter future because of a darker past.

Thank you for reading this book. Please take the time to share it with someone facing hardships.

CPSIA information can be obtained
at www.ICGtesting.com
Printed in the USA
BVHW092037251021
619818BV00008B/170